D0766648

easy gluten-free cooking

195   331

By the same author:

Easy Wheat, Milk & Egg-Free Cooking

over 130 recipes plus
nutrition and lifestyle advice

easy gluten-free cooking

NORWICH CITY COLLEGE LIBRARY		
Stock No.	195331	
Class	641.5631 GRE	
Cat.	Proc.	

rita greer

Thorsons

Thorsons

An Imprint of HarperCollins*Publishers*

77–85 Fulham Palace Road,

Hammersmith, London W6 8JB

The Thorsons website address is www.thorsons.com

First published 1978 as

Gluten-free Cooking

Second edition 1983

Third edition 1989

Fourth edition 1995

This edition revised and updated 2001

10 9 8 7 6

© Rita Greer 2001

Rita Greer asserts the moral right to
be identified as the author of this work

A catalogue record for this book
is available from the British Library

ISBN 0 00 710319 0

Printed and bound in Great Britain by
Martins the Printers, Berwick upon Tweed

All rights reserved. No part of this publication may be
reproduced, stored in a retrieval system, or transmitted,
in any form or by any means, electronic, mechanical,
photocopying, storage or otherwise, without the prior
permission of the publishers.

contents

who needs a gluten-free diet?

There are two kinds of people who need to be on a gluten-free diet. One is the coeliac (celiac) and the other is the gluten allergic. The two are completely different conditions although they are often confused with one another.

coeliacs

Up to the middle of the 20th century, the coeliac condition could prove fatal as a gluten-free diet was not used and medicine, drugs or surgery were not the answer. However, it was discovered that a gluten-free diet could control the illness, and today the outlook for the coeliac is good, providing the gluten-free diet is strictly adhered to. Any lapses, however small, can result in a setback with return of symptoms. The diet is for life in more ways than one.

In coeliacs, the small intestine is affected. This is situated between the stomach area and the large intestine, in the lower part of the abdomen. By the time food reaches the small intestine, half way down the food canal, it is ready to be absorbed into the bloodstream. Any waste food is sent on down to the large intestine. The small intestine has a special lining of little fronds (villi). Each frond is covered in tiny 'hairs' (the brush border). As the food, already processed, passes down the small intestine, the

Changes in small intestine in the coeliac (celiac) condition.

Normal

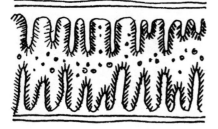

Villi with brush border and particles of food for absorption and digestion.

Abnormal

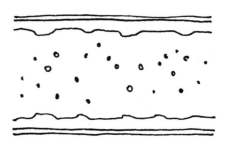

Villi flattened so particles of food cannot be absorbed and digested.

villi and the brush border absorb the nutrients from the food. Unfortunately, in coeliacs, gluten in the food causes the villi to shrink and become quite flattened. The food passes through and fails to be absorbed. This causes unpleasant symptoms and the coeliac becomes malnourished. The patient looks and feels completely 'washed out' – not surprising in the circumstances.

The coeliac condition is a puzzling one to diagnose as the patient seems to eat well but not to thrive. In the case of the coeliac child, there can be failure to grow, and the more the child eats the worse the condition becomes as more gluten is consumed. But there is good news: without gluten in the diet, the damaged lining of the small intestine is able to grow back the villi and brush border. Once the function is restored, health and vitality can be regained and children can grow again.

Some coeliacs with less severe symptoms can remain undiagnosed for years and continually suffer and recover. Common diagnoses for this are a 'digestive disorder', irritable bowel syndrome (IBS), allergy or, worse still, 'imagination'. When eventually diagnosed, it is sometimes called 'silent coeliac disease'.

gluten allergy

The symptoms for food allergy/intolerance/sensitivity are many and varied. They have little or no connection with the coeliac (celiac) condition. An allergy, intolerance or sensitivity to gluten may manifest itself in one or more symptoms. It is difficult to be specific about what is causing the symptoms as they can also be caused by other factors. **People with persistent symptoms should consult their medical practitioner and not try to diagnose and treat themselves.**

physical symptoms

head

Feeling dizzy or faint, headaches, migraine, heavy feeling.

eyes

Watery, itchy, red, swollen, tired, sore, blurred vision, heavy feeling in eyelids.

nose

Runny nose, sneezing, itching, burning, excessive mucus, blocked nose, sinusitis.

ears

Ringing in the ears, soreness, loss of hearing, earache, burning sensations, itching.

throat and mouth

Soreness, sore gums, swollen tongue, mouth ulcers, loss of taste, hoarseness, cough, choking fits, itching of the roof of the mouth, bad breath.

heart and lungs

Chest pains, palpitations, rapid heartbeat, asthma, chest congestion, tightness across chest, shallow breathing, excessive sighing, breathlessness, catarrh.

gastro-intestinal

Nausea, vomiting, stomach cramps, diarrhoea, constipation, swollen stomach, bloated feeling after eating, flatulence, feeling 'full up' long after meals, stomach pains, poor appetite, cravings for foods, dyspepsia.

skin

Rashes, hives, inexplicable bruises, easily marked skin, eczema, excessively pale colour, dermatitis, itching, soreness, redness, sores, acne.

other physical symptoms

Weakness, cramp, cold hands and feet, flushing, shivering fits, trembling, aches and pains in the joints, swelling of the limbs, aches and pains in the muscles, swelling of the face, hands, feet, ankles, constant feeling of hunger, gorging with food, oedema, obesity.

behavioural and psychological symptoms

Nervousness, anxiety, panic attacks, depression, apathy, irritability, day-dreaming, confusion, restlessness, poor concentration, mood swings, aggression, unreasonable giggling or weeping, speech difficulties, couldn't-care-less attitude, general feeling of misery, excessive sleeping, hyperactivity, insomnia.

attitude to a gluten-free diet

The attitudes of both the gluten-free dieter and the rest of the population are crucial concerning the diet. The gluten-free dieter is in a very small minority. The rest of the population forms a huge majority and only a tiny percentage of it has even heard of a gluten-free diet.

getting it wrong

When people feel sorry for a gluten-free dieter it is usually because they perceive the special food to be second-rate in some way and an apology for the real thing. The dieter then feels at a disadvantage and takes on the role of victim, beset with eating problems, always causing a fuss at mealtimes, a burden to the family cook, school meal cooks, family and friends. Food equals a problem, day in, day out. This is a badly managed situation. 'Poor so-and-so, on that dreadful diet.' Disaster!

getting it right

If the special dieter's food looks attractive and tastes good, is interesting and varied the attitude of people around is quite different. They are curious, envious, want taste the food, enjoy it and be on the side of the dieter. This makes the dieter feel special. Problems involving food preparation can be ironed out and so they fade into the background. The dieter is seen to be enjoying food and life. This is a well-managed situation. 'Lucky so-and-so. I wouldn't mind being on your diet.' Success!

cooking skills

Children and adults should be encouraged to take an interest in gluten-free food preparation and be allowed to help in the kitchen. The skill involved is a valuable one for life. It should not be a mystery.

cooking for a gluten-free diet

The sudden introduction of a special diet into the running of a household can be a traumatic experience. Often there is very little help available at the crucial beginning of the diet, especially if there is no dietitian to give advice. If the situation is badly handled the special dieter can unintentionally be made to feel abnormal and a nuisance. A child on a strict diet can instinctively feel he or she is a source of worry as the mealtime routine is suddenly changed.

My advice is don't get into a panic and don't despair. Instead, direct your energy into getting reorganized in the kitchen in order to cope with the new and challenging situation on your domestic front. Millions of people all over the world are in the same predicament, so don't feel you are alone and that the problem is gigantic. It isn't anything that cannot be sorted out easily.

some questions answered

what exactly is gluten?

If you take a teaspoonful of wheat flour and mix it with a little water, the result will be an elastic sort of paste, firmly bound together. The ingredient that makes it bind like this is the *gluten* in the wheat – the 'elastic'. The gluten is actually protein and in a normal diet is a valuable addition. A similar effect is obtained when mixing rye, barley or oat flour with water. Items such as bread can have extra gluten added, as in the so-called 'strong' flours. However, it does not hurt anyone to live without it and millions of people all over the world go the whole of their lives without ever having eaten it, with no ill effects.

where is gluten found?

It is found mainly in wheat, but also in rye, barley and oats. It is only found in *grains* which can be ground into flour. *Note:* There is no gluten in rice although it is an important grain product. There is sometimes confusion about rice which is *glutinous* (different spelling) meaning 'sticky'.

what are wheat, rye, barley and oats used for?

These are mainly used for making bread, cakes, biscuits, pastry and breakfast cereals. Wheat is the most widely used of the four. They are also added to products to thicken them and make them smooth and to help bind them together. For example, they can be put into the sauce that goes with baked beans and into instant puddings.

The flour you buy in the shops for baking is wheat flour, whether plain or self-raising, and the same flour is used in commercial baking for shop bread, cakes, pastries, buns, biscuits etc. Wheat flour is mixed with other grains to give a base for special breads such as rye bread.

are any gluten-free items readily available?

Yes, lots! All fruit and vegetables, meat, fish, pulses, eggs, cheese, milk, yoghurt, butter, cooking oils, rice and nuts are gluten-free, providing they are *plain*.

is gluten-free cooking more difficult than ordinary cooking?

Old fashioned gluten-free cooking was difficult and dull, but the recipes in this book will show you that in most cases it is easier and more delicious than ordinary cooking.

Because manufacturers are not geared to the gluten-free dieter's needs, their labelling can quite inadvertently lead to confusion. If a product lists any of the following substances on the label it may contain gluten, so do check carefully. A good maxim is: *when in doubt, leave it out of your diet.*

flour	rusk
special edible starch	thickening
modified starch	cereal
food starch	binding
corn	cereal protein
starch	binder
cornflour/cornstarch	edible starch
(unless pure)	vegetable protein
thickener	

how can you tell which
commercial products contain gluten?

The following ingredients always contain flour from wheat, rye, barley or oats and therefore are not gluten free:

wheat bran

wheat flour

wheat berries

wheatmeal

wheat flakes

wheat protein

wheat starch (sometimes
  described as special
  gluten-free starch,
  although it is not 100 per
  cent gluten free)

wholewheat

cracked wheat

kibbled wheat

durum wheat

semolina

couscous

wheatgerm

pourgouri

burghul

pinhead oatmeal

oat milk

bulghar/bulgar wheat

granary flour

rye meal

rye flour

rye flakes

barley meal

barley flakes

barley flour

pearl barley

pot barley

oats

porridge oats

rolled oats

jumbo oats

oat flakes

oatbran

oatgerm

oatmeal

'Starch' can mean anything from wheat flour to potato flour. 'Cornflour' can also cover a multitude of sins and can mean all sorts of starches mixed up (UK), unless made purely from maize.

You will find instructions on how to approach manufacturers for information on page 13.

Here is a list of common products likely to contain gluten. Although it is a long list, don't worry! Most of it is 'junk' food and is best avoided in any case.

baby foods*	mayonnaise*
baked beans*	meat with stuffing/coatings
baking powder	muesli
batter and pancake mixes	mustard*
bedtime drinks*	pancakes, pancake mixes
biscuits and biscuit mixes	pastas
blancmange*	paste
breakfast cereals*	pastry, pastry mixes
burgers	pepper (white, catering)
cakes, cake mixes	pickles*
chocolates*	pie fillings
chutney*	porridge
cocoa, drinking chocolate*	potato, instant
coffee (cheap brands)	puddings
communion wafers	salad dressings*
corned beef*	sandwich spreads
cornflour (cornstarch)*	sauces*
cream (non-dairy)	sausages
crispbreads	snacks
crisps (flavoured)*	soups (tinned/packet)
crumble topping	soy sauce*
curry powder*	spaghetti
custard (ready made)*	spreads*

* Check brands to find a possible gluten-free product.

custard powder*	sprouted grains
desserts/instant puddings	stock powder/paste*
fish in crumbs, batter	stuffing
or coatings	suet
gravy powder/mixes	sweets*
ice cream*	yoghurts (flavoured)
macaroni	
malt	* Check brands to find a possible gluten-free product.

For a list of gluten-free products see page 178.

gluten-free?

Legally, manufacturers can label food 'gluten-free' even if it contains a little gluten (UK). This depressing state of affairs is due to an old ruling by the World Health Organization(WHO). Other countries, such as Germany and France, have a more honest 100-per-cent gluten-free standard. The ingredient at the centre of the scandal is wheat starch. This is wheat from which most – but not all – gluten has been processed out with most of its other nutrients. Because it is a waste product it is cheap, and it is the most widely used flour for commercial gluten-free baking. The majority of people who eat it have no idea that it is not truly gluten-free and nor do the people who prescribe it for 'gluten-free' diets.

Rest assured, all the recipes in this book are at the higher 100 per cent gluten-free (of wheat, rye, barley and oats). Wheat starch is not used at all.

are any types of flour naturally free of wheat, rye, barley and oat gluten?

Yes, there are six major ones: ground rice, corn/maize flour (pure cornmeal/cornstarch), potato flour, chickpea flour, millet flour and soya flour. All these are used in the recipes in this book.

how can you find out which products contain gluten?

There are groups specially for people on gluten-free diets who publish lists of gluten-free foods. Unless such groups are enthusiastic, very active, and publish a new list regularly, the lists tend to be outdated and therefore misleading. Another danger is that some organizations may actually be manufacturers and will deliberately ignore products by rival manufacturing companies, thus giving the gluten-free consumer a limited list of products that are available. By being a member of these groups such lists may be made available to you, either free or for a small fee.

You can also approach manufacturers for lists. The best way is to write a straightforward letter, enclosing a stamped addressed envelope, requesting a list of their products which are gluten-free. The larger firms have these lists printed off ready for such enquiries but some firms do not reply on principle. Here is a sample letter to a firm.

Dear Sir or Madam

Gluten-free Products without wheat, rye barley or oats

I am cooking for a gluten-free diet and would be most grateful if you would advise me as to which of your products are gluten-free. I enclose a stamped addressed envelope.

Yours faithfully

It is a good idea to keep a pocket notebook with your own lists of products to avoid. This will prove very helpful when out shopping.

oats and research

In the late '90s, new research in Scandinavia found some coeliacs could tolerate oats. A medical practitioner's advice should be sought before allowing oats in a coeliac's diet. Controversy on the subject goes back many years.

fan ovens – temperature and baking times

As these may vary from one model to another, only guidelines can be given. Generally speaking, temperatures of 20° below those recommended for an ordinary oven and baking times of up to one third less should be effective.

Bear in mind that not all gluten-free foods are necessarily healthy. There are many brands of sweets, confectionery and junk foods available which happen to be gluten-free. By living just on these a health result will not be achieved. See Chapter 14 for help with balancing a gluten-free diet.

the kitchen cupboard

Clear out a particular corner or shelf in your kitchen for the special items you are going to need for baking and cooking. Some of the items you can make for yourself and some you can buy. All of them are suitable for the whole family so don't think it is going to be that difficult to organize.

contamination

One of the problems of gluten-free baking is to avoid contamination by gluten-containing flours such as wheat. It can occur by contact with other items in the kitchen and store cupboard such as wheat flour; by using utensils and equipment which are also used for ordinary cooking, e.g. baking tins; and by airborne means such as flour dust from overalls and aprons. Other dangers are wheat flour under the fingernails and wheat breadcrumbs in the toaster.

If cooking for an acutely allergic person, separate baking tins and utensils are essential. If cooking for a not-so-allergic person, ordinary tins etc. can be used if they are kept scrupulously clean.

gluten-free essentials
for the kitchen cupboard

Black peppercorns

Canned salmon, tuna,
sardines in oil (not sauce)

Chickpea flour*

Cooking oil (sunflower,
soya, corn, olive)

Cornflour (cornstarch)

Dried yeast, instant yeast,
easy blend (check labels)

Fruit juices (pure)

Gelatine crystals

Gram (chickpea) flour*

Ground rice

Honey (pure)

Millet flour*

Potato flour (farina)*

Pure almond and vanilla
flavourings

Rice paper

Sesame seeds

Soft, moist sugars
e.g. demerara

Soy sauce (thin, Tamari-
type, gluten-free brand)*

Spices (ginger, nutmeg,
mixed spice – gluten-free
brand – allspice, ground
cloves, cinnamon etc.)

Sunflower seeds*

Wine or cider vinegar

* Buy from health stores

note

Always check food labels before classing any food as gluten-free. Cornflour (cornstarch) should be pure maize. Some foods will actually be labelled 'gluten-free'.

general items
(Available at supermarkets or grocery stores.)

Bicarbonate of soda

Cooking oils (sunflower,
   soya, extra virgin olive oil)

Cornflour (cornstarch)

Cream of tartar

Fruit juices

Ground rice

Instant yeast/'fast action'
   easy blend yeast

Spices (pure)

Wine or cider vinegar

specialized items
(Probably available at health stores, delicatessens or large chemists/drugstores.)

Rice bran

Gram (chickpea) flour

Maize flour (cornmeal)

Millet flour

Potato flour (farina)

Soya flour

special baking powder

Commercial baking powders are designed to work with gluten, and gluten-containing grains are often used in their manufacture. In a gluten-free diet, special baking powder is required. If you prefer to make your own, here is a recipe:

7g/¼oz/2 tsp	**potassium bicarbonate**
115g/4¼oz/¾ cup	**potato flour (farina)**

Mix these two ingredients together and store in a screw-top jar. Use as required. Try the chemists or drugstore for the first ingredient.

pepper

A word of warning about the use of pepper. It is common practice in commercial catering to add wheat flour to ground white pepper to 'stretch' this expensive commodity. It is therefore a good practice to use only freshly ground black pepper when you are eating out.

margarine

Some 'fancy' margarines have wheatgerm oil added. Check your labels as this is not gluten-free. (Butter is gluten-free.)

soy sauce

Most soy sauces are made from soy beans and wheat so are not gluten-free. Look for *Tamari-type* soy sauce which is made from soy beans and *rice*. This will be gluten-free. Your local health store is the most likely place to find it. Check the label carefully before buying. Get the store to order in several bottles for you. It keeps for years. N.B. Tamari is not a brand name.

gluten-free in a hurry

Just to give you a practical helping hand to start, here are some emergency menus that can easily be followed until you have found sources of the few special ingredients and products you will need for a new and interesting diet.

adults

Eat only the foods specified. They are easily obtainable and most will already be in the store cupboard or refrigerator. Use sea salt and freshly ground black pepper for seasoning. Put polyunsaturated margarine or butter on hot vegetables. Drink tea or coffee with milk. Wine, port, sherry and brandies may be drunk, but no other types of alcohol.

breakfast

- Kellogg's Rice Krispies or Cornflakes (UK), milk and sugar
- Grilled bacon, poached or fried egg, grilled tomatoes, fried mushrooms
- Pure fruit juice

Don't be tempted to eat bread or any other breakfast cereals. If Kellogg's *Rice Krispies* or *Cornflakes* are unobtainable, serve a banana, or add grilled mashed potato to the cooked dish, or make a muesli-type cereal yourself from 1 to 2 heaped tablespoonsful of cold cooked brown rice (boiled the previous day), a sprinkling each of raisins, sesame and sunflower seeds, an eating apple (grated), a little liquid honey to sweeten and milk or fruit juice to moisten.

midday meal

- Boiled or baked potatoes
- Fresh salad of tomatoes, lettuce, cucumber, grated carrot
- Tinned salmon, tuna or sardines in oil or water

Make a dressing from 2 teaspoonsful sunflower oil (or similar), a squeeze of fresh lemon juice, a pinch or two of sugar, sea salt and freshly ground black pepper. If you wish to eat a dessert of some kind, choose any type of fresh fruit – bananas, grapes, apples, oranges, pears etc.

dinner

- Grilled lamb chop, pork fillet or small steak
- Boiled carrots or grilled tomatoes
- 2 plain boiled or steamed green vegetables – cabbage, spinach, French (snap) beans, peas, sprouts etc.
- Plain brown rice, boiled

If you feel the need for a gravy, save the meat juices from the grill pan, strain them off, discard the fat and pour in some of the water strained from the vegetables. Mix well with a wooden spoon and add half a ripe tomato, mashed. Season to taste. Do not use any kind of gravy mix or stock cube/powder.

snacks

Allow yourself up to 3 ripe bananas per day, a few plain almonds or walnuts (English walnuts) and dried fruits such as apricots and raisins.

alternative main meals

Eating out is a problem and best avoided when you start the diet. At home, stick to plain, fresh ingredients and you will have no worries.
Other main meals you might like to choose from are:

- Cold ham (without breadcrumb coating)
- Cold lamb, beef or pork (off a previously roasted joint without stuffing)
- Cold chicken (cooked at home without stuffing) and served with salad and jacket potato
- Roast beef or lamb or pork with roast potatoes (no Yorkshire puddings) served with boiled or steamed vegetables such as carrots, peas, spinach, green beans

emergency ingredients

Without bread, cakes and biscuits (cookies) your starch/carbohydrate intake will be too low. Eat plenty of potatoes and rice to make up for this.

Bear in mind that these are emergency menus and are a little narrow in outlook for a long-term gluten-free diet. However, with this information you should be able to get started immediately rather than continue with an ordinary diet until you have reorganized your eating regime in a broader way. No matter how tempting, *do not eat ordinary bread, cakes, biscuits, crispbreads* etc.

Here is a shopping list/store cupboard check for emergency menus:

- Almonds and walnuts (English walnuts), (plain)
- Bacon
- Black peppercorns
- Brown rice (plain)
- Butter or margarine
- Cooking oil (sunflower or olive)
- Kellogg's Cornflakes or Rice Krispies (if available)
- Dried fruit
- Eggs
- Fresh fruit
- Fresh meat or fish (plain)
- Fresh vegetables
- Milk
- Pure fruit juice
- Salmon, tuna (tunny), sardines – all canned in oil or water (not sauce)
- Sea salt
- Sesame and sunflower seeds (plain)
- Sugar
- Tea or coffee (plain)
- Tomato purée (paste)

emergency menus for children

Use the emergency menus for adults, but omit the alcohol and add extra snacks such as:

- Fresh orange segments sprinkled with a little raw cane sugar;
- Home-made fish cakes *(see page 46)*
- Home-made chips – serve hot with a poached egg on top and grilled tomatoes instead of tomato sauce *(see page 95)*
- Savoury rice – fry a small chopped onion in a little oil. Add chopped cooked vegetables and 1 cup (1¼ cups) of cold cooked brown rice. Heat through while turning over with a wooden spoon. Season and serve
- Milk shakes – blend 2 cups of milk with any piece of stoned, peeled fruit. Add sugar to taste and blend (you will need a blender/liquidizer for this)

staple gluten-free substitutes

basic starchy foods (gluten-free)

As many starchy foods are forbidden on a gluten-free diet, such as ordinary bread, cakes, biscuits, buns, crispbreads, pastas and pizza, etc., other starchy ingredients must take their place in order to maintain a nutritional balance. Rice, potatoes and bananas are all easily available, high in starch and, mercifully, gluten-free. Other such ingredients are tapioca, sago, millet, buckwheat (saracen corn) and kasha, the toasted form of buckwheat. (This commodity is gluten-free in spite of its name, and is a member of the same botanical family as rhubarb.)

potatoes

Potatoes can be cooked in a huge variety of ways and there are always several types on sale all year round, which makes a gluten-free diet more interesting.

Boiled If the potatoes are new, cook them in their skins in boiling, salted water for 20 to 25 minutes, depending on size, until tender. Old potatoes should be peeled and cut into evenly sized pieces first, then cooked for up to 30 minutes, depending on variety.

Mashed Boil old, floury varieties such as King Edwards and Cara until tender, then drain. Mash them in the saucepan with a knob of butter, a little milk and a pinch or two of freshly grated nutmeg, salt and freshly ground black pepper. They can be kept warm for a while in the oven.

Baked (Jacket Potatoes) Scrub old potatoes really well, cutting out any eyes or blemishes. Prick all over with a fork and bake for an hour in an oven preheated to 425°F/220°C/gas mark 7 or for 2 hours at 350°F/180°C/gas mark 4. Cut open and insert a knob of butter to serve. Leftover baked potatoes can be sliced, including skin, and fried in a little sunflower or olive oil the following day.

Roast Potatoes Peel old potatoes and cut into even-sized chunks. Place in a roasting tin and sprinkle with 1 tsp sunflower or olive oil for each medium-sized potato. Turn over by hand to coat the potato chunks with the oil, then roast at the top of the oven for about ¾ hour on a high heat or 1 hour on a medium heat until crisp, golden and tender.

Chips (French Fries) Many brands of oven chips are not gluten-free, so it is safer to make your own (*see page 95*).

Potato Spaghetti A useful, quick way to cook potatoes, especially for breakfast as they only take 10 minutes (*see page 110*).

Potato Patties Peel old potatoes, then boil and mash them. Season to taste. Form into small balls, then flatten and shallow fry in a little hot olive oil or sunflower oil until crisp and golden. Drain on kitchen paper and serve.

Potato flour (farina), available from health stores, is useful for coating foods before frying and for thickening gravies, stews, casseroles and sauces.

rice

Rice is widely available and there are many varieties. Serve basmati rice with curries and use other varieties for puddings and savoury dishes. Boil in plenty of water. The cooking time depends on the hardness of the grains, and varies from 10 to 15 minutes for basmati to 45 minutes for brown rice. When the rice is tender, drain through a colander and serve. Keep it hot, if necessary, by placing the colander over a pan of simmering water, covering with a saucepan lid or plate and just leaving until required. To reheat rice, put it into a metal sieve over a pan of water and bring to the boil. Steam for a few minutes, until hot.

Ground and flaked rice are good additions to the kitchen cupboard for a gluten-free diet. Rice flour is more finely ground than ground rice but is not easy to come by. Flaked rice is used for puddings.

buckwheat (saracen corn)

This is not from the wheat family and does not contain gluten. It is cooked in the same way as rice. Kasha is the toasted form of buckwheat and tastier than the plain kind. Buy from health stores and cook in the same way as rice. Buckwheat flour has rather limited uses but can be made into pancakes successfully. Buy from health stores.

cornflour

True cornflour (cornstarch) is finely ground maize/sweetcorn. Always check that the label specifies maize, as sometimes other grains are added that are not gluten-free.

cornmeal

This is a coarse form of ground corn on the cob (maize) and can be used to make *cornbread (see page 35)*.

millet

A gluten-free, creamy coloured product sold as flakes or flour. The flakes can be ground to flour in a coffee grinder (electric). Buy at health stores.

gram (chickpea flour)

This looks yellow and smells rather like peas. It is useful in giving gluten-free baking an attractive colour. Buy at health stores.

The more you can rely on cheaper staples, such as potatoes and rice, for the carbohydrates (starch) in a gluten-free diet, the cheaper the diet will be and the fewer expensive substitutes you will need. Pulses such as beans and lentils are starchy foods but many gluten-free dieters have difficulty digesting them. However, if they do not present a problem they are a good addition to the diet.

bread

There is one very important food around which a gluten-free diet revolves. This is bread, and life without it can be difficult; there is no way to fill the gap left by wheat bread other than to substitute another kind that is just as nutritious and versatile. In this chapter there are recipes for gluten-free breads and other baked items which are easy to make and comfortably fill this gap.

active dried yeast (granules)

This is not mixed into the flour like Easyblend (instant) yeast. It needs to be mixed with warm water and allowed to swell before adding to the flour. If you are using this type of yeast, take some of the water from the recipe, warm it and sprinkle in the yeast with the sugar. Leave it in a warm place until frothy, then stir and add to the flour with the rest of the liquid. Please note that brewer's yeast is not suitable for baking.

homemade pectin for binding

Without gluten, baking disintegrates into crumbs. This is the most difficult problem that has to be solved for gluten-free baking. To some (and only some) extent, doughs and mixtures can be bound together with grated apple, pectin, egg white and mashed potato.

Dried pectin is extremely difficult to obtain and very expensive. Liquid pectins are available for jam setting but are not suitable for baking. However, it is very easy to make your own pectin for gluten-free cooking from something you normally throw away.

Whenever you peel a cooking apple, save the peelings. Wrap and store in the freezer to use when required.

Put the peel from 1 medium cooking apple into a small saucepan. Cover with a teacup of water and bring to the boil. Cook without covering for about 15 minutes or until the liquid has reduced to about 6 tbs. Strain through a wire mesh sieve, pressing the peelings with the back of a wooden spoon and saving the strainings in a basin. Discard the skin and put the strainings to one side to cool. When cold it will be like a thin jelly, pale green in colour.

Use as directed in the recipes but putting in 2 tbs of the pectin to start with. After mixing it into the batter, if it feels too thin, add the remaining tbs of pectin and it will thicken as you stir. Obviously, the strength of the pectin depends on the apple and how much pectin you manage to extract in the cooking.

easy crusty bread

No need to let this loaf wait before baking as it will rise in the oven.

makes one small loaf

170g/6oz	**potato flour (farina)**
30g/1oz	**gram (chickpea) flour**
30g/1oz	**cornflour (cornstarch)**
¼ tsp	**salt**
1 level tsp	**sugar**
7g/¼oz	**instant yeast**
1 tbs	**sunflower oil**
2–3 tbs	**homemade pectin** *(see page 29)*
125ml/4fl oz/½ cup	**lukewarm water**

1 Preheat oven to 350°F/180°C/gas mark 4.

2 Grease a 500g/1lb small loaf tin.

3 Put the flours, salt, sugar and yeast into a bowl. Mix well, teasing out any lumps with the fingers.

4 Add the oil, pectin and water. Mix/beat to a thick, creamy batter.

5 Pour/spoon into the prepared tin and put on the top shelf to bake for 50 minutes to 1 hour until well risen, golden and with a cracked top.

6 Turn out onto a wire rack to cool as soon as it comes out of the oven. Do not cut until cold as the loaf needs to 'set'.

7 Eat freshly baked or the following day toasted/fried. Use any leftovers for breadcrumbs. Keep wrapped in cling film to prevent drying out.

note to cooks   Avoid squeezing the loaf when freshly made as this will make cracks inside.

easy sesame loaf

This bread will rise during baking so does not need to be left to prove. The carrot increases the fibre content.

170g/6oz/1 cup	**ground rice**
30g/1oz	**cornflour (cornstarch)**
30g/1oz	**gram (chickpea) flour**
7g/¼oz sachet	**instant yeast**
¼ tsp	**salt**
½ tsp	**sugar**
30g/1oz	**finely grated carrot (fresh)**
2–3 tbs	**homemade pectin** *(see page 29)*
1 tbs	**sunflower oil**
140ml/5fl oz/⅔ cup	**lukewarm water**
	sesame seeds for topping

1 Preheat oven to 350°F/180°C/gas mark 4.
2 Grease a 500g/1lb small loaf tin.
3 Put the ground rice, flours, yeast, salt and sugar into a bowl. Mix well.
4 Add the carrot, pectin and oil and mix again.
5 Stir in the water and mix/beat to a thick batter.
6 Turn into the prepared tin, level the top with a knife and sprinkle with sesame seeds. Put immediately into the oven and bake on the top shelf for 50 minutes to 1 hour.
7 Turn out of the tin and cool on a wire rack. Leave to grow cold before cutting. Eat freshly baked or toasted the following day.
8 Keep wrapped in cling film to prevent drying out.

pizza dough

This will give you enough dough for 1 medium-sized pizza or 3 small ones for starters or snacks.

30g/1oz	**millet flour (see note below)**
30g/1oz	**cornflour (cornstarch)**
60g/2oz/⅓ cup	**ground rice**
2 good pinches	**bicarbonate of soda**
3 good pinches	**cream of tartar**
1 good pinch	**salt**
30g/1oz	**polyunsaturated margarine**
30g/1oz	**mashed potato (fresh)**
about 4 tbs	**milk**

1   Put the first 6 (dry) ingredients into a bowl and mix well.
2   Rub in the margarine and then the mashed potato.
3   Add enough milk to mix to a stiff paste. Knead into 1 ball of dough.
4   Use immediately for pizza. See pages 93 and 172 for instructions and toppings.

note to cooks   Millet flakes can be ground in a coffee grinder to make flour.

dropscones

Use instead of bread on the day they are made. A useful recipe as it doesn't require an oven.

makes twelve

15g/½oz	**millet flour**
30g/1oz	**cornflour (cornstarch)**
70g/2½oz	**ground rice**
3 good pinches	**cream of tartar**
2 good pinches	**bicarbonate of soda**
2 level tsp	**caster sugar**
1	**egg, beaten**
60ml/2fl oz/¼ cup	**milk**
	sunflower oil for greasing

1   Put a griddle or heavy-based frying pan to heat on the hob.
2   Mix the millet, cornflour (cornstarch), ground rice, cream of tartar, bicarbonate of soda and sugar into a bowl.
3   Stir in the egg.
4   Pour in the milk and mix/beat to a creamy batter.
5   Put a little oil into a saucer. Use a screw of kitchen paper to lightly grease the hot pan, and turn the heat down to medium.
6   Stir the batter. Drop tablespoons of it into the pan. These will spread out into circles. Cook until bubbles appear then turn over with a spatula and cook on the other side for a minute.
7   Stack on a warm plate. Serve freshly made, covered with a cloth napkin to keep them warm.

cornbread

This is a soft bread that can be served with a spoon – hence its alternative name, spoonbread – and is popular in the USA, where corn is a staple. It makes a good side dish but is not suitable for sandwiches or toast, and is best served warm from the oven. Cornmeal (not to be confused with cornflour/cornstarch) is available from health stores, Indian grocers and some supermarkets.

1 tbs	**sugar**
¼ tsp	**salt**
3 tsp	**gluten-free baking powder** *(see page 17)*
160g/6oz/1½ cups	**cornmeal**
50g/2oz/½ cup	**rice flour or ground rice**
1	**egg**
300ml/½ pint/1¼ cups	**skimmed milk**
1 tbs	**sunflower oil**

1 Preheat the oven to 425°F/220°C/gas mark 7.
2 Put the sugar, salt, baking powder, cornmeal and rice flour into a bowl and stir to combine.
3 Beat the egg with the milk in a basin and stir in the oil. Add to the cornmeal mixture and stir well until you have a smooth batter.
4 Pour into a 23cm/9 in. pie dish that has been well greased with sunflower oil and bake on the top shelf of the oven for 30 to 35 minutes, until beginning to brown.
5 Serve straight from the oven in large spoonfuls or cut into wedges.

flatbread

An unyeasted giant scone to bake quickly, as required.

30g/1oz	**millet flour**
30g/1oz	**cornflour (cornstarch)**
60g/2oz/⅓ cup	**ground rice**
¼ level tsp	**bicarbonate of soda**
½ tsp	**cream of tartar**
3 good pinches	**salt**
30g/1oz	**polyunsaturated margarine**
30g/1oz	**fresh mashed potato**
4 tbs	**milk**

1   Preheat the oven to 425°F/220°C/gas mark 7.
2   Thoroughly mix the 6 dry ingredients in a bowl.
3   Rub in the margarine and then the potato.
4   Stir in the milk and mix to a stiff paste.
5   Put onto a greased baking sheet and shape by hand into a large, round scone.
6   Use a sharp knife to cut a cross on the top and bake for 15 to 20 minutes until golden.
7   Cut into wedges, split and spread with polyunsaturated margarine or butter.

chapattis

makes two large

45g/1½oz	**ground rice**
15g/½oz	**gram (chickpea) flour**
15g/½oz	**cornflour (cornstarch)**
2 good pinches	**salt**
5 tbs	**cold water**
	sunflower oil for greasing

1 Put the ground rice, gram flour, cornflour and salt into a basin. Mix well.

2 Add the water and stir with a tablespoon to make a thin cream. Transfer to a jug.

3 Heat a heavy-based frying pan. Using kitchen paper, grease the pan lightly with a little oil.

4 Pour in half the mixture, tilting the pan to allow it to spread into a circle. Cook over a steady heat for about 2 minutes then turn the chapatti over, loosening it with a spatula. Cook on the other side, pressing it flat with the spatula to speed up the process.

5 Serve stacked on a plate to tear into pieces for eating with curry or salads. Eat freshly made.

poppadoms

Make as for chapattis but finish in a hot oven for about 10 minutes to make them crisp and crunchy.

note to cooks   The batter should be thin enough to run when the pan is tilted. If left to stand, the batter will thicken and require more water to obtain the correct consistency.

pancake batter

makes four small or two large pancakes

45g/1½oz	**ground rice**
15g/½oz	**cornflour (cornstarch)**
pinch	**salt**
1	**egg**
140ml/¼ pint/⅔ cup	**milk**

1 Mix the ground rice, cornflour and salt in a bowl.
2 Beat the egg in a cup and pour into the flour mixture. Mix with the fork.
3 Add about ⅓ of the milk. Beat in with the fork until it is absorbed and there are no lumps. Gradually add the remaining milk and beat to a thin, smooth cream.
4 Transfer to a jug.

pancakes

Pancakes are a useful bread substitute in a gluten-free diet. They can be filled with sweet or savoury fillings and are suitable to eat at any time of day.

batter *(see page 39)*
sunflower oil

1 Heat a pancake pan or heavy-based frying pan. Grease with a screw of kitchen paper dipped in a little oil.
2 When the pan begins to smoke, pour in enough batter for 1 pancake. Tilt the pan so that the batter completely covers it. Cook for about a minute and the edge begins to brown. Use a spatula to loosen it and turn the pancake over to cook on the other side for a minute.
3 Keep warm in the oven on a warmed plate while you make the remainder, whisking the batter each time before pouring and greasing the pan again.
4 Use for fruit pancakes for breakfast or a pudding, or for savoury pancakes for a main meal.

scones

Ideal for breakfast, as a snack or for tea.

makes two large or four small

15g/½oz	millet flour
15g/½oz	cornflour (cornstarch)
60g/2oz/⅓ cup	ground rice
2 good pinches	bicarbonate of soda
3 good pinches	cream of tartar
1 heaped tsp	caster sugar
15g/½oz	polyunsaturated margarine
30g/1oz	fresh mashed potato
	milk to bind

1 Preheat oven to 425°F/220°C/gas mark 7.
2 Mix the first 6 (dry) ingredients in a bowl.
3 Rub in the margarine and then the mashed potato.
4 Stir in enough milk to bind and mix to a smooth, stiff dough.
5 Break the dough into 2 or 4 pieces. Shape each one into a round scone.
6 Place on a greased baking sheet and bake for 15 minutes on the top shelf for the large ones and about 12 minutes for the small ones.
7 Cool on a wire rack. Serve freshly baked, to split and butter.

golden crispbreads

These look so inviting everyone will want one – deliciously light, crisp and golden.

makes five large

45g/1½oz	**ground rice**
15g/½oz	**cornflour (cornstarch)**
15g/½oz	**gram (chickpea) flour**
2 good pinches	**salt**
3 good pinches	**caster sugar**
20g/¾oz	**polyunsaturated margarine**
30g/1oz	**fresh mashed potato**
2 tsp	**water**

1 Preheat oven to 425°F/220°C/gas mark 7.

2 Mix the ground rice, cornflour, gram flour, salt and sugar in a bowl.

3 Rub in the margarine, then the mashed potato.

4 Add the water and mix by hand to a smooth dough, kneading lightly for a few seconds.

5 Divide into 6 equally sized pieces.

6 Grease a baking sheet. Put a piece of dough onto it and roll with a straight-sided tumbler or mini rolling pin into a thin circle about 10.5cm/4 in. in diameter. Do the same with the remaining 5 pieces.

7 Prick all over with a fork and bake for 10 minutes on the top shelf until crisp and golden. Leave to cool on the baking sheet or put immediately into a basket. Eat freshly baked with meals instead of bread.

note to cooks   Do not move the crispbreads after rolling out on the baking sheet because they will be too thin and fragile.

sesame crispbreads

Make as for Golden Crispbreads but before baking, sprinkle lightly with sesame seeds and roll to press them into the surface.

breakfasts

rice porridge

This is good for cold winter mornings. Follow with grilled bacon and special gluten-free bread *(see pages 30 and 32)* fried on one side in hot vegetable oil.

¼ litre/½ pint/1⅓ cups	**milk**
2 tbs	**ground brown rice**
2 tsp	**vegetable oil**
1 tbs	**sultanas/golden seedless raisins or**
	chopped dried apricots
2 heaped tsp	**sugar**
15g/½oz/2½ tbs	**ground almonds**

1   Put the milk and ground rice into a saucepan and stir until smooth.
2   Add the oil and dried fruit and heat to boiling point. Cook over a medium heat, while stirring with a wooden spoon, for a few minutes until the porridge thickens and the fruit swells. Take off the heat.
3   Add the sugar and almonds. Stir well and serve hot.

fish cakes

These fish cakes can be made in advance, stored in the fridge and fried as required. Do not keep for more than 36 hours before using.

makes about six

¼ kilo/½ lb/1¼ cups	**cooked fish such as haddock, cod or coley**
¼ kilo/½ lb/1 cup	**cold, boiled potato**
25g/1oz/2½ tbs	**polyunsaturated soft margarine**
1 heaped tbs	**freshly chopped parsley**
	sea salt and freshly ground black pepper
	sunflower oil for frying

1 Mash the fish with the potatoes and the margarine.

2 Add the remaining ingredients and mix well with a fork until the fish and parsley are evenly distributed.

3 Form into round, flat cakes with the hands.

4 Fry in hot, shallow oil for 3 minutes on each side or 4 minutes if the fish cakes have been in the fridge.

5 Serve immediately with grilled tomatoes and special gluten-free bread (*see Easy Crusty Bread, page 30*) and margarine or butter.

variation   Tinned salmon or tuna (in water or oil) may be used instead of white fish. (Drain well before using.)

As alternatives to just plain frying, try dipping the fish cakes in cornflour (cornstarch) and beaten egg then roll them in special gluten-free breadcrumbs before frying; or brush them with milk and dip them in special gluten-free breadcrumbs.

note to cooks   Commercially-made fish cakes often use wheat-bread crumbs as a coating.

special breadcrumbs

Break slices of special gluten-free bread into pieces. Grind to crumbs in a coffee grinder (electric).

muesli

1–2 tbs	suitable base – cold cooked rice
1	ripe eating apple, washed and sliced
½	ripe banana (optional), sliced
1 tbs	raisins
1 tbs	chopped nuts
1 tsp	sesame seeds
1 tsp	sunflower seeds
	diluted fruit juice or milk
	brown sugar to taste (optional)

1   Put all the ingredients into a cereal bowl.
2   Pour over juice or milk and serve.

note to cooks   Other dried fruits can be used such as chopped dried apricots or peaches, stoned prunes etc. If fresh fruit is not available, soaked dried fruit salad can be used for variation. To save time, a basic muesli of dry items can be made, stored in an air-tight jar and used as required. This way more variety can be achieved.

muesli base

50g/2oz/⅓ cup	raisins
75g/3oz/⅔ cup	chopped nuts – walnuts, cashews, Brazils, etc.
50g/2oz/⅓ cup	sesame seeds
75g/3oz/¾ cup	sunflower seeds
25g/1oz/¼ cup	ground almonds
50g/2oz/⅓ cup	chopped dried apricots
50g/2oz/⅓ cup	chopped stoned prunes

1 Combine all the ingredients.
2 Store in an air-tight jar and use as required.

note to cooks   Use as a base with fresh fruit, sugar or liquid honey to taste and milk to moisten.

toasted muesli

Put 1 heaped tbs chopped hazelnuts and cashew nuts into a sponge tin. Place under a hot grill for a minute. Stir and sprinkle in 1 tsp sesame seeds. Grill again until golden brown. Use with the remaining ingredients, as for Muesli.

potato and beans

	vegetable oil for frying
2	**baked or boiled potatoes, cut into slices**
1 portion	**gluten-free baked beans in tomato sauce**

1 Put a little oil in the frying pan and heat for a few seconds. Add the potato slices and cook on both sides until golden and crisp.

2 At the same time, heat the beans gently in a small saucepan.

3 Serve at once on a warmed plate.

note to cooks   The potatoes can be cooked the day before, either baked in their skins or boiled in salted water. Use a gluten-free brand of baked beans such as Heinz. Check the label before using.

beans on toast

Toast thick slices of gluten-free bread (*see pages 30 and 32*). Spread with poly-unsaturated soft margarine and top with hot gluten-free baked beans in tomato sauce.

bubble and squeak

Heat a little oil in a frying pan, then fry leftover greens and potato (pre-cooked and chopped up) made into a little cake. When browned, turn and fry the other side. Season with sea salt and freshly ground black pepper. Serve hot with grilled bacon.

kedgeree

Although this sounds a rather strange dish for breakfast, it was a popular item on the menu for the Victorian breakfast table as it made use of the leftovers of the previous day.

serves one

2–3 heaped tbs	**cooked brown rice**
50g/2oz/⅓ cup	**cooked, flaked haddock or cod**
1	**medium-sized tomato, chopped small**
1	**egg, hard-boiled**
	sea salt and freshly ground black pepper
	vegetable oil

1 Mix together the first three ingredients and season.
2 Heat a little oil in a saucepan. Add the rice mixture and heat thoroughly while stirring gently. Top with chopped hard-boiled egg.
3 Season and serve hot on a warmed plate.

breakfast platter

50g/2oz/1 small piece	**lamb's liver or kidneys**
	gluten-free cornflour
2 slices	**back bacon**
2 slices	**special gluten-free bread**
2	**medium-sized tomatoes**

1 Wash the liver or kidneys and cut out any strings or white bits, then cut into slices.
2 Dip the slices in flour (cornstarch) and fry in a little hot vegetable oil.
3 At the same time, put the bacon, bread and tomatoes under a hot grill, turning the bread over to toast both sides.
4 Serve on a warmed plate with the tomatoes on the toast.

variation   Fry 3 or 4 sliced mushrooms with the liver.

fruit pancakes

makes one serving

Make the pancakes as on page 40. Spread with jam, sweetened stewed fruit or fresh fruit and roll up. Dust with caster sugar and serve on a warm plate. Choose a filling from the following:

Jam – strawberry, raspberry, blackcurrant, black cherry

Stewed fruit – apple, apple and raspberry, blackberry and apple, plum, greengage, plum and apple, mixed fruit, summer fruits, summer fruits and apple, peaches, apricots, peach and raspberry, apricot and apple

Fresh fruit – mashed raspberries, sliced strawberries, chopped blueberries, chopped peaches, mashed banana

Canned fruit – peaches, apricots, pears, fruit salad, de-stoned prunes

Traditional lemon – allow ¼ lemon per pancake. Squeeze juice all over each pancake with a sprinkle of caster sugar and roll up. Also use orange or a mixture of orange and lemon

Golden syrup or runny honey – drizzle from a tablespoon over the pancake and roll up. No caster sugar required for serving.

breakfast pizza

serves one

	pizza dough *(see page 33)*
2–3	(canned) peeled plum tomatoes, chopped
2	rashers back bacon, trimmed of fat
2	eggs
	polyunsaturated margarine
	milk

1 Preheat oven to 425°F/220°C/gas mark 7.
2 Make the pizza dough as instructed on page 33.
3 Put the dough onto a greased ovenproof plate. Press out with the fingers into a circle about 15cm/6 in. in diameter. Raise an edge all round.
4 Cover the base with the chopped tomatoes and put into the oven for 15 minutes on the top shelf.
5 While the base is baking, grill the bacon and chop into small squares. Scatter over the tomatoes.
6 Put a small knob of margarine into a small pan and add 1 tbs milk. Heat gently to melt the margarine. Add the egg, breaking it up with a wooden spoon as it cooks and sets. While still soft and creamy, take off the heat.
7 Spread over the pizza and serve piping hot. Season to taste.

other breakfast suggestions

cheese on toast with tomatoes

Toast slices of special gluten-free bread (*see pages 30 and 32*) on both sides. Cover one side with thin slices (or grated) Cheddar cheese. Grill for a minute. Put slices of tomato on the cheese and continue grilling until the cheese is bubbly and the tomato cooked.

bacon and egg

Grill slices of back bacon. Serve with a poached egg on special gluten-free toast (*see pages 30 and 32*).

cowboy's breakfast

Serve slices of grilled bacon with hot gluten-free baked beans in tomato sauce on special gluten-free bread (*see pages 30 and 32*) or with fried, cold boiled potatoes.

scrambled egg and tomato

Serve 2 eggs scrambled with a little milk on special gluten-free toast *(see pages 30 and 32).* Garnish with grilled tomatoes or fried mushrooms.

boiled egg and toast fingers

Lightly boil an egg (3 or 4 minutes). Serve with fingers of buttered special gluten-free bread, toasted.

omelette filled with fried mushrooms

Make an omelette with 2 eggs. Fill with 50g/1oz mushrooms, fried in a little sunflower oil or similar.

note to cooks   To top up any of these, serve a gluten-free cereal, milk and brown sugar or special gluten-free toast, butter and marmalade.

snacks

Snacks may be an important feature of a diet for those who experience a sudden weight loss when they change over from an ordinary diet to a gluten-free one. As all fruit (fresh) is gluten-free, what could be more simple than a piece of fruit as a snack? Bananas are particularly useful and should be regarded as a staple food.

The following recipes are for both sweet and savoury snacks. Biscuits and cookies can be baked in batches and stored in air-tight containers to be used as required. Don't make the mistake of storing biscuits and cookies together as the cookies, being moist, will soften the biscuits. Any biscuits which do go soft in storage can easily be recrisped in the oven for a few minutes.

sandwiches

As most commercial spreads contain gluten, you will need to fall back on home-made spreads and sandwich fillings. One consolation about this situation is that at least you will know exactly what you are eating!

Use special gluten-free bread *(see pages 30–32)*, cut thinly and spread with margarine on one side. Spread one slice or lay on a filling and press the other slice on top. Cut off the crusts for a luxury sandwich. Open sandwiches need only the bottom slice of bread and can be decorated or garnished to look attractive. Unless very easy to manage, serve these with a knife and fork.

fillings/spreads

Always make freshly as you need them. Wrap individually in cling film to keep them moist for a lunchbox.

1   Cottage cheese and chopped dates (not too many) – this makes a very moist sandwich.
2   Hard-boiled egg, chopped and mixed with cress or watercress, finely chopped. This will give you a pale green filling which looks more interesting than most other spreads. Season with sea salt and black pepper.
3   Tinned fish (in oil), drained and mashed with chopped hard-boiled egg and a little tomato purée (paste), or gluten-free mayonnaise.
4   Thin slices of tomato, seasoned with sea salt and a little black pepper, sprinkled with a little sugar and a few chopped chives.

hot jam sandwich

This is rather like a giant doughnut and looks and tastes delicious. For each sandwich you will need two slices of fairly thick gluten-free bread *(Easy Crusty Loaf, page 30)*, margarine, jam (jelly) and caster sugar.

Heat margarine in a frying pan and fry each slice of bread on one side only, until crisp and golden. Sprinkle a little caster sugar on a warm plate and lay one of the slices on it, fried side down. Spread with jam (jelly) and cover with the other slice of bread so that the fried side is uppermost. Sprinkle with a little more sugar and serve right away with a spoon.

hamburgers

makes two

100g/4oz/⅔ cup	lean minced beef
1 thin slice	special gluten-free bread *(see page 30)* made into crumbs
1 small	egg, beaten
	sea salt and freshly ground black pepper
scant tsp	gluten-free soy sauce
½	small onion, finely chopped
	ground rice
	olive oil for frying

1 Put all the ingredients, except the rice and oil, in a basin and mix well.
2 Shape the mixture by hand into 2 flat cakes.
3 Dip the burgers in the ground rice to give a thin coating.
4 Fry in a little hot oil, turning once, for 3 to 4 minutes on each side.
5 Serve with low-fat chips *(see page 95)* and grilled tomatoes.

note to cooks   These can be made in advance and stored in the fridge between two plates for a few hours until required. If you don't have any special gluten-free bread for crumbs, use 1 heaped tablespoon of cooked rice (chopped) or cold mashed potato.

cookies

As most commercial biscuits are made with wheat, you will need to make your own at home.

spiced currant cookies

makes eight to ten

50g/2oz/¼ cup	**polyunsaturated soft margarine**
100g/4oz/½ cup	**ground rice**
75g/3oz/1 small	**eating apple, finely grated**
40g/1½oz/¼ cup	**demerara sugar**
½ tsp	**gluten-free mixed spice**
40g/1½oz/¼ cup	**currants**

1 Preheat oven to 450°F/230°C/gas mark 8.

2 In a bowl, blend the margarine and ground rice with a fork.

3 Add the apple, sugar, spice and currants. Knead and mix with a wooden spoon until one large ball of dough is formed.

4 Grease a baking sheet and put 8 to 10 spoonfuls of the dough on to it. Spread out into cookie shapes with a knife.

5 Bake for about 20 to 25 minutes.

6 Allow the cookies to cool on a baking sheet, then remove them with a spatula and allow to cool on a wire rack. (The cookies will go crisp as they cool down.)

note to cooks Eat within 48 hours of baking.

nut brownies

makes six

1	egg white
65g/2½oz/½ cup less 1 tbs	sugar
65g/2½oz/½ cup plus 1 tbs	ground nuts – almonds, hazelnuts, walnuts
	or mixed nuts
1 tbs	ground rice
½	orange, grated rind of
	rice paper

1   Preheat oven to 350°F/180°C/gas mark 4.
2   Whisk the egg white until stiff.
3   Stir in the sugar and nuts.
4   Fold in the ground rice and orange rind.
5   Use a tablespoon to place 6 rounds on a baking sheet lined with rice paper, with plenty of space between them.
6   Bake on the centre shelf for 20 to 25 minutes.
7   Remove from oven, allow to grow almost cold and then take them off the baking sheet.
8   Trim the surplus rice paper with kitchen scissors.

ginger spice cookies

Light, melt-in-the-mouth cookies to hand round and make people envious.

makes twenty-four

115g/4oz/⅔ cup	**ground rice**
55g/2oz	**cornflour (cornstarch)**
½ level tsp	**bicarbonate of soda**
1 level tsp	**ground ginger**
3 good pinches	**ground cloves or mixed spice**
30g/1oz	**polyunsaturated margarine**
30g/1oz	**soft brown sugar**
1 rounded tbs	**golden syrup**
½	**egg, beaten**

1　Preheat oven to 350°F/180°C/gas mark 4.

2　Mix the ground rice, cornflour, bicarbonate of soda and spices in a bowl.

3　In a separate bowl, beat the margarine to a cream.

4　Add the sugar and cream again.

5　Beat in the golden syrup and the egg.

6　Add the dry mixture from the first bowl. Mix well to make a soft, sticky paste.

7　Put heaped teaspoons of the mixture onto a greased baking sheet, leaving plenty of space around each one, flattening them with the back of the teaspoon.

8　Bake for about 12 minutes on the top shelf.

9　Lift off gently with a spatula and leave to cool and crisp on a wire rack. Store in an airtight container, individually wrapped in cling film.

note to cooks　　If this mixture turns out too soft, mix in a little more cornflour (cornstarch).

apricot and cinnamon cookies

makes four

25g/1oz/2½ tbs	**gluten-free soft margarine**
50g/2oz/½ cup	**ground rice**
½	**eating apple, finely grated**
1 tbs	**brown sugar**
6	**dried apricot halves, chopped**
3 pinches	**cinnamon**
	sunflower oil for greasing
2 tsp	**sesame seeds**

1 Preheat oven to 450°F/230°C/gas mark 8.

2 In a bowl, use a fork to blend the margarine and ground rice.

3 Add the apple, sugar, apricots and cinnamon. Mix with a wooden spoon until the dough forms 1 ball.

4 Grease a baking sheet with the oil. Divide the dough into 4 portions and put on the greased baking sheet, spreading each portion out with the back of a teaspoon to make a cookie shape. Sprinkle each one with ½ teaspoon sesame seeds and press them in slightly.

5 Bake above centre of oven for 20 to 25 minutes. Cool on the baking sheet for 2 to 3 minutes then lift the cookies off with a spatula. Leave to cool and grow crisp on a wire rack.

6 Eat within 24 hours of baking.

nibbles

Most party or cocktails titbits contain gluten so you will need to make your own. It is perhaps easier to make up little dishes with naturally gluten-free items rather than spend ages in the kitchen baking up curious items!

Here is a list of possibles: radishes, small whole tomatoes, spring onions (scallions) – for non-sensitive tummies, celery stalks, all kinds of nuts, sunflower seeds, raisins, dried apricots and sultanas (golden seedless raisins). Remember: all fresh fruit is gluten-free.

cheese nibbles

makes twelve crisp little biscuits

30g/1oz	ground rice
15g/½oz	pure cornflour (cornstarch)
1 level tbs	finely grated Parmesan cheese
1 heaped tsp	polyunsaturated margarine
½	egg, beaten
¼ tsp	gluten-free French mustard

1   Preheat oven to 400°F/200°C/gas mark 6.
2   Put the ground rice, cornflour and cheese into a basin. Mix well.
3   Add the margarine and rub in until the mixture resembles crumbs. Stir in the egg and mustard. Mix to a smooth paste.
4   Break off small pieces of the paste, about the size of a small walnut. Put onto a greased baking sheet and spread out with the back of a teaspoon into small circles. Texture each one with a fork, pressing the prongs to make a pattern.
5   Bake for 8 to 10 minutes until pale golden brown. Put on a wire rack to cool. Serve with drinks or as a snack nibble. Store in an airtight container and use within a week.

note to cooks   Genuine French mustard will be gluten-free as the French do not allow thickening in their mustards.

soups and starters

Home-made soups are always far superior to the commercial ones. Serve as a snack or with a meal. Pack in a vacuum for picnic meals.

Traditional soup recipes may not need any alterations to make them gluten-free. Take care with thickenings and stock. Do not add any kind of noodles unless gluten-free (special) ones. Use freshly ground black pepper instead of white pepper.

split pea soup

serves three to four

¼ kilo/½ lb/1 cup	**dried split peas**
1 large or 2 small	**onions, peeled and sliced**
1 tbs	**vegetable oil**
½ litre/1 pint/2½ cups	**water**
1 tbs	**Tamari-type gluten-free soy sauce**
¼ kilo/½ lb/8oz	**carrots, trimmed, scrubbed and sliced**
	sea salt and freshly ground black pepper

1   Put the split peas into a fine mesh sieve and wash them under the cold tap.
2   Put the peas into a large bowl with well over ½ litre/1 pint of water and leave overnight to swell.
3   Fry the onion in the oil for 3 or 4 minutes. Pour in the fresh water and the soy sauce.
4   Strain the soaked peas and add them to the saucepan with the carrots and a sprinkling of salt. Bring to the boil and lower heat, simmering gently with the lid on for 1 to 1¼ hours, stirring from time to time. (If the soup thickens too much, add more water.)
5   Season to taste and serve hot.

note to cooks   This is a very nourishing and filling soup. Serve with gluten-free bread (*see pages 30 and 32*) or special sippets (*see page 77*).

winter vegetable soup

seves three to four

1	medium-sized onion, peeled and sliced
1 tbs	thin vegetable oil
1	medium-sized carrot, scrubbed and sliced thinly
1 small	parsnip, peeled and sliced
1 small	turnip, peeled and sliced
4	sprouts, trimmed and sliced
1	medium-sized potato, peeled and sliced
½ litre/1 pint/2½ cups	water
1 tbs	Tamari-type gluten-free soy sauce
	sea salt and freshly ground black pepper

1 Fry the onion in the oil.
2 Put in the rest of the vegetables and about half the water.
3 Bring to the boil and then simmer with the lid on for about 20 minutes.
4 Add the rest of the water to cool it down, then liquidize.
5 Return the soup to the pan, heat through and add the soy sauce and seasoning to taste.
6 Serve hot.

variation   Just before serving, add 1 heaped tablespoonful of freshly chopped parsley.

mulligatawny soup

Make as for Winter Vegetable Soup. Add 1 level tsp gluten-free mild curry powder with the onion and crush in 1 glove garlic. Stir in well before serving.

cream of mangetout soup

serves two

½	medium onion, chopped
1 tbs	sunflower oil
100g/4oz/¼ lb	mangetout (snow peas), trimmed and cut up
½	small potato (for thickening), peeled and sliced
425ml/¾ pints/2 cups	water
2–3 tsp	gluten-free soy sauce
	salt and freshly ground black pepper
4 tsp	single (light) cream (dairy)

1 In a saucepan, fry the onion gently in the oil for 5 minutes or until soft and transparent; do not let it brown.

2 Add the mangetout (snowpeas), potato slices, water and soy sauce. Cover the pan and bring to the boil. Lower the heat and simmer for about 12 to 15 minutes.

3 Remove the pan from the heat and leave until the soup has cooled slightly. Blend in a liquidizer, then pour back into the pan and season to taste. Reheat gently, then serve with 2 teaspoons of cream swirled into each bowl of soup.

celery soup

serves two

½	medium onion, peeled and sliced
2 tsp	thin vegetable oil
2–3	stalks of celery, including leaves, washed and chopped small
150ml/¼ pint/⅔ cup	water
2 scant tsp	Tamari-type gluten-free soy sauce
	sea salt and freshly ground black pepper

1 Fry the onion gently in the oil until transparent.

2 Add the celery and stir-fry with the onion for 3 to 4 minutes.

3 Liquidize with the water.

4 Pour the soup back into the saucepan, bring to the boil, then simmer for 5 minutes.

5 Pour into a jug and strain back into the saucepan through a fine mesh sieve.

6 Add the soy sauce and seasoning.

7 Leave to stand for a few hours, then reheat and serve.

parsley soup – cold

serves three

1	small onion, peeled and sliced thinly
1 tbs	vegetable oil
2	medium-sized potatoes, peeled and sliced thinly
50g/2oz/2 cups	fresh parsley, washed and chopped
3 tsp	Tamari-type gluten-free soy sauce
½ litre/1 pint/2½ cups	water
	sea salt and freshly ground black pepper

1 Fry the onion in the oil for 3 to 4 minutes with the lid on.
2 Add the potato slices and chopped parsley. Stir and add the soy sauce and water. Bring to the boil and simmer with the lid on for half an hour.
3 Remove from the heat and allow to cool for a few minutes. Liquidize in a blender and return to the saucepan.
4 Taste and season. Dilute with more water if you think it is too thick.
5 Allow to cool. Pour into a jug and place in the fridge for at least an hour. Serve cold from the fridge.

watercress soup

serves three

1	medium-sized onion, peeled and sliced thinly
2 tsp	vegetable oil
1	medium-sized cold boiled potato
1 bunch	watercress (including stems), washed thoroughly and coarsely chopped
400ml/¾ pint/2 cups	water
2–3 tsp	Tamari-type gluten-free soy sauce
	sea salt

1   Fry the onion in the oil until transparent but not brown.
2   Put the onion, potato, watercress and about half the water into the liquidizer and blend until smooth. Pour into the saucepan.
3   Add the remaining water and the soy sauce. Bring to the boil and simmer for 10 minutes.
4   Season to taste and serve hot or cold.

onion and tomato soup

serves two to three

2	medium-sized onions
25g/1oz/2½ tbs	polyunsaturated soft margarine
1	400g/14oz tin tomatoes
1 tsp	sugar
2 tsp	Tamari-type gluten-free soy sauce
	sea salt and freshly ground black pepper

1 Fry the onion in the margarine until transparent.
2 Liquidize the tomatoes with the cooked onion and return to the saucepan.
3 Add the sugar, soy sauce and seasoning.
4 Bring to the boil and simmer while stirring.
5 Serve hot, diluted with water if preferred.

mushroom soup

serves two

½	medium-sized onion, peeled and sliced thinly
2 tsp	vegetable oil
50g/2oz/1 cup	fresh mushrooms, washed and sliced
¼ litre/½ pint/1⅓ cups	water
1–2 tsp	Tamari-type gluten-free soy sauce
	sea salt and freshly ground black pepper

1 Fry the onion in the oil for 3 to 4 minutes.
2 Place the fried onions, mushroom slices, water and soy sauce in a liquidizer. Blend and pour back into the saucepan.
3 Bring to the boil and simmer for about 5 minutes.
4 Season to taste and serve hot.

sippets

Lightly fry cubes of special gluten-free bread in hot vegetable oil until golden. Sprinkle into hot soup and serve. (Cut the bread into thick slices and then into cubes.)

hot grapefruit

When the rest of the family eats something different, it is useful to have a quick recipe for the gluten-free dieter as a starter.

½ grapefruit serves one person

½   **grapefruit**

sugar

polyunsaturated soft margarine

1   Loosen the flesh of the grapefruit all round with a sharp knife, and also cut between the segments.
2   Place the grapefruit in the grill pan and sprinkle with a little sugar.
3   Put a small knob of the special margarine in the centre and grill for 2 to 3 minutes until it begins to brown and bubble.
4   Serve immediately in a rounded bowl with a teaspoon.

liver pâté

serves five to six

¼ kilo/½ lb/8oz	chicken livers
	sea salt and freshly ground black pepper
1	small onion or shallot, peeled and chopped very finely
1 tbs	sunflower oil
3 good pinches	dried mixed herbs
1	small clove of garlic, peeled
1 tsp	sherry or white wine

1 Wash the livers and cut out the stringy parts and yellow pieces.
2 Dry thoroughly and chop into small pieces. Sprinkle with salt and pepper.
3 Fry the chopped onion in the oil for 3 to 4 minutes, using a small saucepan.
4 Add the chopped liver and herbs, and crush in the garlic through a garlic press.
5 Turn up the heat a little and stir with a small wooden spoon. The liver will start to crumble and turn a pinky-brown colour. This should take about 5 minutes. Mash with a fork to a smooth paste.
6 Add the sherry or white wine. Stir, taste and correct seasoning.
7 Allow the pâté to cool, then place it in little dishes and cover with a foil lid. Store in the fridge and eat within 3 days.
8 Serve with hot gluten-free toast or as a spread in sandwiches made with gluten-free bread (*see page 30*). Garnish with parsley.

note to cooks   Unsuitable for pregnant women.

crudités

Served with dips such as special mayonnaise *(see page 82)*, these make an ideal starter.

Radishes – scrubbed and trimmed.

Celery – scrubbed and trimmed and cut into short lengths.

Carrot – washed and trimmed and cut into matchstick shapes.

Spring Onion (Scallion) – washed and trimmed.

Cauliflower – use the crisp, white florets after washing well.

Lettuce – use just the heart leaves. Wash and pat dry with a clean tea-towel. (Any variety of lettuce will do.)

Tomato – only use if you can get small fruits. Wash and leave whole.

Fennel – cut white part into matchsticks.

Courgettes – cut into small sticks, leaving the skin on.

Red and green peppers (Bell peppers) – cut into short slices after taking out the stem and seeds.

prawn cocktail

Another useful starter to serve to the gluten-free dieter when the rest of the family is eating something else.

serves one

1	lettuce leaf
½	medium-sized tomato
25g/1oz/2½ tbs	peeled prawns
1 tbs	egg mayonnaise *(see page 82)*
½ tsp	tomato purée/paste
4 or 5 drops	lemon juice
3 or 4 pinches	sugar
	sea salt and freshly ground black pepper
	parsley sprigs to garnish

1 Tear the lettuce leaf into small pieces and put into a glass dish.
2 Cover with the tomato, cut into wedges.
3 Place the prawns on top.
4 Put the mayonnaise into a cup with the tomato purée (paste) and mix.
5 Add the lemon juice and the sugar. Stir well.
6 Taste and season with salt and pepper. Pour or spoon the dressing over the prawns. Garnish with the parsley.

egg mayonnaise

Commercially produced mayonnaise often contains gluten. Make your own at home and enjoy a gourmet experience. Use extra virgin olive oil (cold pressed) for best results, or sunflower oil if you prefer something less robust in flavour.

makes just over 285ml/½ pint/1⅓ cups

300ml/½ pint/1¼ cups	**extra virgin olive or sunflower oil**
1	**egg**
1	**egg yolk**
2 tbs	**wine vinegar**
½ tsp	**gluten-free mustard (genuine French mustard will be suitable – look for 'made in France' on the label)**
3 pinches	**salt**
	freshly ground black pepper

1 Have all ingredients ready at room temperature. Measure out the oil in a jug.

2 Put the egg, egg yolk, 1 tablespoon of vinegar, mustard and salt into a liquidizer and blend for a few seconds.

3 With the motor running, slowly add the oil a few drops at a time. When about half the oil has been used you can increase the rate at which you add it.

4 Add the remaining tablespoon of vinegar and switch off. If the mayonnaise is too thick, stir in a little boiling water (about 1 tablespoon). Do not switch on the liquidizer to incorporate it.

5 Spoon the mayonnaise into a scrupulously clean screwtop jar and label and date it. Store in the fridge and use as required but throw away any remaining after 2 weeks.

note to cooks   The vinegar increases the pH sufficiently to act as a deterrent for salmonella bugs. Although this should make this raw egg sauce safe it is prudent for pregnant women, children and older people not to use this type of cold, uncooked sauce – just in case.

mushrooms à la grecque

serves four

1	medium-sized onion, grated
2 tbs	sunflower oil or similar
1 wineglass	dry white wine
1	small clove garlic, peeled
350g/¾ lb/6 cups	button mushrooms
4	medium-sized fresh tomatoes
	sea salt and freshly ground black pepper
	chopped fresh parsley

1 Fry the onion in the oil for 3 to 4 minutes, but do not let it brown.

2 Add the wine and crush in the garlic through a garlic press.

3 Wash the mushrooms and leave them whole.

4 Stab each tomato with a fork and plunge into boiling water. As they split, remove and peel them. Cut into quarters.

5 Put the mushrooms and tomato quarters into the onion mixture. Cook for about 10 minutes until the liquid has halved in quantity.

6 Season to taste and leave to grow cold. Chill in the fridge and serve in small dishes with a sprinkling of parsley. At the same time, serve fingers of special gluten-free toast and margarine or butter.

variation   If you do not want to make this with white wine, use a non-fizzy kind of apple juice instead.

suggestions for other starters

Melon.

Fresh grapefruit with a little sugar.

Mixed grapefruit and orange segments with a little sugar.

Avocado with prawns and egg mayonnaise *(see page 82)*.

Radishes or tomatoes with special gluten-free bread and butter.

Green salad of lettuce (2 kinds), watercress, cucumber, green pepper strips etc. Sprinkle
with 3 pinches of sugar, sea salt and freshly ground black pepper, 2 teaspoonfuls
of sunflower oil and 1 teaspoonful of wine vinegar. Serve in individual bowls.

main meals

egg florentine

serves one

100g/4oz/½ cup	**cooked and well drained spinach, chopped small**
15g/½oz/1 tbs	**butter**
	grated nutmeg
	sea salt and freshly ground black pepper
1	**egg**
1 tbs	**Parmesan cheese, grated**

1 Heat the spinach with the butter and sprinkle with a couple of pinches of nutmeg.
2 Put into a small ovenproof dish and make a hollow in the middle.
3 Carefully break the egg into the hollow and sprinkle the cheese over it.
4 Bake in a preheated oven at 350°F/180°C/gas mark 4 for about 15 minutes or until the egg is set.
5 Serve with toasted special gluten-free bread (*see pages 30 and 32*).

note to cooks   Can also be served as a poached egg on top of cooked spinach, without the cheese.

baker's omelette

This recipe makes enough for 3 or 4 servings, so can be served to the whole family. A very quick and nourishing meal.

serves three to four

1	small onion, peeled and chopped
1 tbs	sunflower oil
2	boiled potatoes, sliced
2	tomatoes
2	medium-sized mushrooms
1 heaped tbs	cooked peas or chopped cooked vegetables
6	eggs
	sea salt and freshly ground black pepper
1 tsp	chopped fresh parsley

1 Preheat oven to 450°F/220°C/gas mark 7 and put in a largish, shallow, ovenproof dish to warm on the top shelf.
2 Fry the onion in the oil for about 5 minutes.
3 Add the vegetables and gently heat through.
4 Transfer to the warmed dish.
5 Beat the eggs in a bowl and season.
6 Pour over the vegetables and bake on the top shelf for about 10 to 15 minutes until the eggs have set.
7 Sprinkle with the chopped parsley and serve hot with a side salad.

chicken with orange and rosemary

serves two

2	chicken quarters, or breasts, skinned
3 pinches	salt
	freshly ground black pepper
1 tbs	extra virgin olive oil (mild flavoured) or sunflower oil
1	onion, sliced
225ml/8fl oz/1 cup	orange juice
½ tsp	dried rosemary or
1 tsp	fresh
1	small orange, grated rind of
2 slightly heaped tsp	gluten-free cornflour cornstarch, mixed to a paste with
2 tsp	cold water

1 Season the chicken all over with salt and pepper and rub in.

2 Heat the oil in an ovenproof casserole and fry the chicken pieces for about 7 to 8 minutes, turning them over to brown evenly.

3 Remove the chicken from the pan, add the onion and fry gently, stirring, for 5 minutes.

4 When the onion is soft, add the orange juice, rosemary and orange rind.

5 Put the chicken pieces back into the casserole and bring to the boil, then reduce the heat and simmer gently for about 30 minutes, until the chicken is tender. Transfer the chicken to a warmed serving dish and keep warm.

6 Stir the cornflour (cornstarch) paste into the liquid and bring to the boil. Cook, stirring for 2 minutes until it has thickened, then pour it over the chicken.

7 Serve hot with boiled rice and green beans or a green salad.

cottage pie

Either serve to the family or cook ahead and freeze for the gluten-free dieter.

serves four

2	medium-sized onions, sliced
2 tbs	vegetable oil
½ kilo/1 lb	lean, minced beef
1 tbs	ground brown rice
1 heaped tsp	tomato purée/paste
3 tsp	Tamari-type gluten-free soy sauce
150ml/¼ pint/⅔ cup	water
	sea salt and freshly ground black pepper
4 portions	hot, boiled potatoes
25g/1oz/2½ tbs	polyunsaturated soft margarine
	a little water
3 pinches	grated nutmeg

1   Preheat oven to 375°F/190°C/gas mark 5 and put a casserole in to warm.

2   Fry the onion in the oil for about 5 minutes.

3   Add the beef and fry very gently while stirring for another 5 minutes.

4   Sprinkle in the ground rice and add the tomato *purée* (paste) and soy sauce.

5   Stir well and add enough water to make a sloppy mixture.

6   Season and spoon into the warmed casserole. Put back into the oven to keep warm.

7   Mash the potatoes well, adding the margarine.

8   Pour in a little water and beat with a wooden spoon.

9   Add the nutmeg and season to taste. Give it a final stir and pile on top of the meat mixture, spreading it out evenly over the top with a fork.

10   Bake for about 30 minutes on the middle shelf, then serve hot with green vegetables and carrots.

note to cooks   Put into 4 suitable dishes and freeze until required. Defrost slowly and heat thoroughly before eating.

spanish omelette

A good quick meal that makes the minimum of washing-up! Some people prefer it without the pepper (green or red) as they find it rather indigestible.

serves one

1 tbs	vegetable oil
1	medium-sized boiled potato, cut into thick slices
1	small onion, sliced finely
small piece	green or red pepper, cut into strips
2	medium-sized tomatoes, sliced
½	small clove garlic, peeled
2	eggs
1 tsp	cold water
	sea salt and freshly ground black pepper

1 Put the oil into a heavy-based frying pan.
2 Heat the potato slices and the onion.
3 Fry, turning once, for about a minute on each side.
4 Add the strips of pepper and the tomatoes. Crush in the garlic and distribute it in the pan.
5 Beat the eggs lightly with the water and when you think the pan is hot enough, pour over the cooked mixture. Cook for about 4 minutes or until the eggs have set.
6 Season to taste and loosen the omelette with a spatula. Serve immediately cut in wedges on hot plates with a green side salad.

main meal pizza

A useful dish for when the rest of the family is eating something different. Served with a green salad and fruit it makes a complete meal. For a really large pizza, double the ingredients and make it 23cm (9 in.) in diameter.

serves one

170g/6oz	**pizza dough** *(see page 33)*
3	**canned, peeled plum tomatoes, chopped**
1 slice	**ham (without breadcrumb coating),** **cut into small squares**
1 medium	**mushroom, chopped**
1 heaped tsp	**chopped fresh parsley or basil**
1 tbs	**finely chopped onion**
1	**stick celery or courgette (zucchini), sliced thinly**
1 heaped tbs	**finely grated tasty Cheddar cheese**

1 Preheat oven to 425°F/220°C/gas mark 7.

2 Put the dough in the centre of a greased baking sheet. Press out with the fingers to a circle about 15cm (6 in.) in diameter. Raise an edge all round to keep the filling in place.

3 Cover with the chopped tomatoes and scatter the ham squares over.

4 Sprinkle over the mushroom and herb followed by the onion. Cover with the celery or courgette (zucchini), top with the cheese and bake on the top shelf for about 15 minutes.

5 Serve hot with a green side salad.

plaice with cucumber

serves one

1	**fillet of plaice**
1 tbs	**ground brown rice mixed with**
2 pinches	**sea salt**
25g/1oz/2½ tbs	**polyunsaturated soft margarine**
squeeze	**lemon juice**
3.5cm/1½in	**cucumber, peeled and cut into thick slices**

1 Put a dinner plate to warm.

2 Wash the plaice fillet and coat with the rice.

3 Put the margarine into a frying pan, heat and use to fry the plaice, turning once. This should take about 4 minutes.

4 Take the pan off the heat and remove the fish with a spatula. Put on to the warmed plate and keep warm.

5 Add the lemon juice to the pan, stir and return to the heat.

6 Add the cucumber slices and quickly heat through. Arrange them on top of the fish.

7 Serve immediately with carrots, grilled tomatoes or any brightly coloured vegetables and plain boiled brown rice.

note to cooks   Seasoning is put on at the table.

fish and chip dinner

Going to someone else's house for a meal can be a nightmare for the gluten-free dieter and the host or hostess who wants to help but doesn't understand the diet. Here is an easy main meal within the capabilities of any cook. You may need to take your own gluten-free cornflour (cornstarch) or some ground rice, just to make sure.

serves one

2	**medium-sized potatoes**
2 tbs	**extra virgin olive oil or sunflower oil**
1	**egg white**
2 tsp	**gluten-free cornflour (cornstarch) or ground rice**
100–160g/4–6oz	**portion of plain cod or haddock**
2	**tomatoes, halved**
2 heaped tbs	**frozen peas**

1   Preheat the oven to 450°F/230°C/gas mark 8.
2   Peel the potatoes and cut them into chips (French fries). Put them in a roasting tin (pan) with 2 teaspoons of the oil and turn them over by hand to coat them.
3   Roast on the top shelf of the oven for about 20 to 25 minutes.
4   After 15 minutes, beat the egg. Dip the fish in cornflour (cornstarch) to coat and then in the egg. Arrange the tomato halves in a small ovenproof dish and put into the oven on the bottom shelf.
5   Put the peas on to cook in boiling water. Heat the remaining oil in a frying pan and fry the fish over a moderate heat for 5 minutes. Carefully turn it over and cook the other side.
6   Serve on a warm plate with the chips, tomatoes and peas.

lamb with herbs

serves one

1 or 2	lamb chops
1	clove garlic
	dried rosemary
	sea salt and freshly ground black pepper

1 Trim the chops of fat and wash them under the tap. Dry and put into the grill pan on a grid.
2 Cut the clove of garlic in half and rub over the meat.
3 Sprinkle with a little rosemary and seasoning.
4 Grill for about 15 minutes, turning once.
5 Serve at once with gravy (*see page 98*), boiled potatoes and hot green vegetables. Peas and carrots are especially good with this dish.

lamb with redcurrant jelly

Grill lamb chops on a grid for about 15 minutes, turning once. Serve hot with redcurrant jelly, hot vegetables, mashed potatoes and gravy *(see page 98)* to which you have added 1 heaped tsp redcurrant jelly.

gravy

Many people believe that gravy can only be made with a stock/gravy cube or a packet mix. This is nonsense. The best gravy is made from the natural stock contained in meat juices, a little thickening such as maize flour (cornmeal) and the strainings from vegetables. A little Tamari-type gluten-free soy sauce can be added for colouring and extra flavour. See page 18 for details of suitable soy sauce.

1   Strain the fat off the meat juices from the grill or roasting pan.
2   Sprinkle in about 1 to 2 heaped teaspoonsful of maize flour (cornmeal) and rub it into the juices with a wooden spoon.
3   While you heat, gradually add the strainings from any vegetables you have cooked, and 1 to 2 teaspoonsful of Tamari-type gluten-free soy sauce.
4   Stir while it thickens and serve hot with the meat and vegetables. If it turns out lumpy, then strain before using.

variation   Use half a boiled and well mashed potato as a thickener instead of the maize flour (cornmeal).

note to cooks   It is important to strain off all the fat from the meat juices or the gravy will be far too greasy.

liver with orange

serves one

50g/2oz/ 1 medium-sized piece	**lamb's liver**
1 tbs	**vegetable oil**
½	**peeled orange, cut into slices**
2 tsp	**Tamari-type gluten-free soy sauce**
1 tbs	**pure orange juice**

1 Cut out any stringy pieces from the liver. Wash, dry and cut it into small pieces.
2 Heat the oil in a frying pan and put in the liver. Fry gently while turning to cook evenly for 5 minutes.
3 Add the orange slices, soy sauce and orange juice. Heat through gently.
4 Serve hot with green vegetables and either plain boiled brown rice or potatoes.

variation   If you prefer a thicker gravy, dip the liver pieces in maize flour (cornmeal) before frying. (Seasoning is added at the table.) Unsuitable for pregnant women.

cold meat and salads

Beef, lamb and pork slices cut off a cold joint roasted the day before make an easy meal with salad and jacket potatoes. Here are some salad suggestions. Instructions for the jacket potatoes are on page 26.

red salad

The colour of this salad is simply amazing! Serve with plain, cold roast chicken or pork and jacket potatoes.

serves four

75g/3oz/½ cup	**red pepper, cut into strips**
150g/6oz/1 cup	**red cabbage, shredded**
100g/4oz/1 cup	**carrot, grated**
100g/4oz/1 cup	**fresh tomato, chopped**
100g/4oz/1 cup	**raw beetroot, grated**

1 Wash and prepare the vegetables.
2 Cut the red pepper into strips.
3 Shred the red cabbage finely.
4 Grate the carrot.
5 Cut the tomato into small pieces.
6 Grate the beetroot coarsely.
7 Combine all the ingredients in a bowl and dress lightly before serving with an oil and vinegar dressing and a seasoning of sea salt and black pepper.

variation   For a slightly sweet salad sprinkle a little sugar over the finished salad. (This is especially good with cold pork or ham.)

green salad

There are several types of greens, other than lettuce, that can be used for a green salad. Any mixture of the following on a base of either lettuce or cabbage will make an excellent salad.

Watercress – washed very carefully. Discard tougher stems and any discoloured leaves. Tear into sprigs.

Cress or Mustard Greens – cut off as near to the roots as you can and rinse in a colander under the cold tap.

Cabbage – choose heart leaves that will not be too tough. Wash and trim coarse stalks away. Shred finely.

Spinach – use young, tender leaves. Cut out coarse stalks. Tear the leaves into small pieces.

Kale – use only tender leaves. Wash well and tear or cut into small pieces.

Brussels Sprouts – trim, wash and shred finely.

Lettuce – wash leaves well and pat dry with a clean tea-towel. Tear into pieces.

Rocket – wash leaves and tear into pieces.

Sliced spring onions (scallions) or the ordinary type of onion (chopped or sliced into rings) can also be used in a green salad; cucumber and finely chopped fresh parsley also make useful garnishes. Serve with an oil and vinegar dressing, but first sprinkle the mixed salad with a few pinches of sugar, sea salt and freshly ground black pepper.

oil and vinegar dressing

Put 1 tablespoonful of wine or cider vinegar and 3 tablespoonsful sunflower oil and 1 level teaspoonful caster sugar (optional) into a screw-top jar. Shake well before using. (This dressing should be used to moisten salads not to swamp them.)

stir-fry vegetables

This is a quick method of partly cooking vegetables so that they are just soft enough to eat. Use a large flat pan with sloping sides. Prepare a mixed selection of vegetables, cutting them into small pieces or thin slices (root vegetables). Always start with a sliced onion and a tablespoonful of sunflower oil. Stir while you fry this for 3 minutes. Now add the rest of the vegetables in order of hardness, carrot first, cucumber and tomato last. As you put them in, use the middle of the pan and keep turning them over. Push the cooked vegetables to the side of the pan and the raw ones into the middle. Add a sprinkling of sea salt and a tablespoonful or two of water. Mix a little Tamari-type gluten-free soy sauce with the juices and you have a lovely gravy. What could be easier?

savoury rice

serves two

1	medium-sized onion, peeled and chopped
1 tbs	sunflower oil
½	green pepper, de-seeded and chopped
1	carrot, scrubbed and chopped
1	stalk of celery, washed and chopped
3	Brussels sprouts or
2	tender cabbage or spinach leaves, shredded after trimming
1 portion	cooked brown rice
	sea salt and freshly ground black pepper to taste
	squeeze of lemon juice (optional)

1 Fry the onion gently in the oil for a few minutes.
2 Add the prepared vegetables and a little water to prevent sticking.
3 Cook with the lid on tightly for about 6 to 7 minutes.
4 Add the cooked rice and mix everything together. Cook until the rice has heated through.
5 Season and add the lemon juice, if liked.
6 Serve hot with fish or meat.

variation   Other kinds of vegetables can be used according to season – green beans, peas, turnips, parsnips, broad beans (Windsor beans) etc. If you want to use tomato this is best served as a garnish as it is very soft when cooked and tends to make the dish too moist.

rice with mushrooms

A simple but very tasty dish.

serves two

½	medium-sized onion, chopped
	sunflower oil
2	medium-sized mushrooms, chopped
1 portion	cooked brown rice
1–2 tsp	Tamari-type gluten-free soy sauce
1 tbs	single cream
	salt and freshly ground black pepper

1 Fry the onion in 2 tsp sunflower oil until soft and transparent.

2 Fry the mushrooms in 1 tbs sunflower oil for 2 to 3 minutes.

3 Combine the onions and mushrooms and mix with the cooked brown rice and soya/soy sauce.

4 Add the single cream and season to taste.

5 Serve hot with grilled steak or pork and a green side salad.

basic savoury sauce mix

1 tbs	**butter or margarine**
15g/½oz/1 tbs	**gluten-free cornflour (cornstarch)**
¼ litre/½ pint/1⅓ cups	**milk**
	flavouring from list *(see page 107)*
	sea salt and freshly ground black pepper

1　Melt the margarine in a saucepan.

2　Blend the maize flour (cornmeal) and milk in a bowl, stirring out any lumps.

3　Pour this into the pan with the margarine and stir well.

4　Add the flavouring of your choice.

5　Heat through and simmer for about 3 minutes, stirring all the time while the mixture cooks.

6　Serve hot, immediately, on fresh vegetables or fish.

note to cooks　Make sure the cornflour (cornstarch) is gluten-free.

flavourings

Parsley – add 1–2 level tsp chopped fresh parsley.

Mushroom – add 50g/2oz fried mushrooms, chopped very finely.

Onion – add one small onion, fried in a little sunflower oil until soft. Chop the onion very finely before frying.

Tomato – add 1 tbs tomato purée (gluten-free). Stir in well.

Cheese – add 25–50g/1–2oz/¼–½ cup grated hard cheese or Parmesan cheese. Cook the sauce while stirring until all the cheese has melted.

Watercress – add 2 heaped tbs chopped watercress leaves. (Good with baked salmon.)

Serve any of these savoury sauces poured over baked, poached or steamed fish. Serve with a green vegetable such as peas and potatoes or rice, plain boiled.

cauliflower cheese

Pour hot cheese sauce over plain boiled or steamed cauliflower. Sprinkle a little more cheese on top and brown under the grill for a few minutes. The cauliflower should be tender but not soft as this will spoil the dish. Serve with special gluten-free bread (*see pages 30 and 32*) and butter or margarine.

leeks in cheese sauce

serves one

1 medium	**leek**
1	**hard-boiled egg**
	cheese sauce
	grated cheese for topping

1 Cook the leek, cut into short lengths, in boiling salted water until tender.
2 Strain well and put into an ovenproof dish.
3 Peel the hard-boiled egg. Slice and lay on top of the leek.
4 Cover with cheese sauce.
5 Sprinkle with grated cheese and grill until bubbling and just beginning to brown.
6 Serve hot with special gluten-free bread *(see pages 30 and 32)* and butter or margarine.

potato 'spaghetti'

serves one

2	medium-sized potatoes, peeled
1 tsp	olive or sunflower oil for greasing pan

1 Preheat the oven to 425°F/220°C/gas mark 7.
2 Thinly slice the potatoes lengthways and then cut them into long matchsticks. Place in a greased baking tin (baking pan).
3 Bake on the top shelf of the oven for 10 minutes, until tender but not crisp.
4 Serve in a mound, covered with a gluten-free sauce *(see page 111)*.

sauce for potato 'spaghetti'

serves one

¼	onion, finely chopped
1 scant tbs	olive oil
1 slice	lean ham (without breadcrumbs), cut into small squares
2	tomatoes, chopped
½ tsp	tomato purée (paste)
1	mushroom (chopped)
¼ tsp	dried basil or
½ tsp	chopped fresh basil
	salt and freshly ground black pepper
1 tbs	Parmesan cheese, finely grated

1 Fry the onion in the oil for 4 minutes. Add all the remaining ingredients except the cheese and cook, stirring, for another 5 minutes.

2 Spoon the sauce over the Potato 'Spaghetti' *(see page 110)* or boiled rice and sprinkle with the cheese. Serve hot with a green salad or lightly cooked spinach or broccoli.

bolognese sauce

four generous servings

1	medium-sized onion, peeled
1 tbs	sunflower oil
1	clove garlic, peeled
4	small mushrooms, chopped
100g/4oz	lean, minced (ground) beef
½	small green pepper, de-seeded and chopped
4	medium-sized tomatoes, sliced
1 tbs	Tamari-type gluten-free soy sauce
	sea salt and freshly ground black pepper

1 Chop the onion and fry gently in the oil for about 4 minutes until transparent.
2 Add the minced (ground) beef and fry lightly, turning it over with a spatula until cooked.
3 Put in the garlic (crushed), mushrooms, peppers and tomatoes.
4 Mix and season with the soy sauce and salt and pepper.
5 Heat through and cook for about 10 minutes while you stir.
6 Serve hot on boiled rice or potatoes or potato spaghetti.

note to cooks   This can be re-heated the following day. Store overnight in the fridge, in a sealed container.

baked fish

serves one

1	portion cod, haddock or salmon fillet
	sea salt and freshly ground black pepper to taste
½	lemon, juice of
1	orange, rind of
	small knob of butter

1 Preheat oven to 375°F/190°C/gas mark 5.
2 Put the fish in a shallow ovenproof dish and season.
3 Pour the juice over the fish and sprinkle with the rind.
4 Dot with butter and bake uncovered for about 15 minutes near the top of the oven.
5 Serve immediately with stir-fry vegetable or savoury rice (*pages 103 and 104*). Garnish with a sprinkling of parsley and a slice of lemon.

note to cooks   Salmon cooked this way is especially good with plain boiled new potatoes and broccoli florets. Garnish with lemon and parsley.

baked salmon with watercress sauce

serves one

1	**fresh salmon steak**
juice of ½	**lemon**
	salt and freshly ground black pepper
2 slightly rounded tsp	**cornflour (cornstarch)**
1 heaped tbs	**low-fat dried milk granules**
140ml/5fl oz/⅔ cup	**water**
handful	**watercress leaves, chopped**

1 Preheat oven to 350°F/180°C/gas mark 4.

2 Place the fish in a greased shallow ovenproof dish. Squeeze over the lemon juice and season to taste.

3 Cover with a double thickness of greased, greaseproof paper and bake for 20 minutes on the top shelf.

4 Put the cornflour, milk granules and water into a small saucepan. Heat through gently while stirring. Bring to the boil and simmer for 2 minutes until thickened.

5 Stir in the watercress. Allow to cool for a few minutes then spoon into a liquidizer. Blend to a bright green sauce. Season to taste.

6 Serve the salmon on a warm plate with the hot sauce spooned partly over it and partly on the plate. Garnish with a sprig of watercress and a twist of lemon. Serve with boiled new potatoes, peas and sliced carrots or broccoli.

date and apple chutney

2	cooking apples, grated coarsely
2	medium-sized onions, finely chopped
6 tbs	wine vinegar
2 heaped tbs	chopped, de-stoned dates
2 heaped tbs	soft brown sugar

1   Put the apple, onion and vinegar into a medium saucepan. Cook/stir over a medium heat until the mixture is soft.
2   Stir in the chopped dates and cook for another 2 minutes.
3   Add the sugar and mix well. Bring to the boil then take off the heat.
4   Put into a jar and leave to grow cold.
5   When completely cold, cover with cling film and store in the fridge.
6   Use as required with cold meat, cheese, for sandwiches and with curry.

note to cooks   For extra flavour, 3 pinches of allspice can be added with the sugar.

chinese stir fry

Over-spiced food and a gluten-free diet seldom go together. The exotic elements in this recipe are restricted to just ginger and garlic. For the meat, use raw chicken breast, pork fillet, rump or sirloin steak, cut into wafer thin strips across the grain of the meat to ensure it will be tender when cooked. Use a wok or large, shallow-sided saucepan to cook this quick, tasty meal.

serves two

115g/4oz/½ cup	**raw meat strips**
2 heaped tsp	**cornflour (cornstarch)**
1 tbs	**Tamari-type gluten-free soy sauce**
55g/2oz	**green fine beans**
5	**salad onions (scallions)**
½	**red pepper**
1 tbs	**sesame oil**
1 heaped tsp	**finely chopped fresh ginger**
1 small	**clove garlic, finely chopped**
115g/4oz/1⅓ cups	**fresh beansprouts**
2 tbs	**sherry**
1 tbs	**water**
2 portions	**boiled, long-grain rice, to serve**

1   Put the meat strips into a basin with the cornflour and soy sauce. Mix well and leave to marinate while you prepare the vegetables.

2   Trim the beans and cut into short lengths. Trim the roots off the onions and the coarsest green off the tops. Cut remainder into short lengths, making diagonal cuts. Cut out the stem and seeds from the pepper and discard. Cut the flesh into thin strips.

3   Heat the oil in a wok. Stir-fry the marinated meat with the ginger and garlic for 3 to 4 minutes over a medium heat.

4   Add the beans, onion and pepper. Stir-fry for 4 minutes then put in the beansprouts and continue for another minute.

5   Spoon in the sherry and water and cover the pan with a lid for a minute to steam the beansprouts.

6   Serve with hot, boiled rice on warm plates.

curried eggs with almonds

Vegetarian and not too spicy.

serves two

½	medium-sized onion, chopped finely
1 tbs	sunflower oil
1 tsp	finely chopped fresh ginger
1 level tsp	mild curry powder (gluten-free brand)
1	medium-sized carrot, sliced thinly
1	small potato, sliced thinly
2 tsp	Tamari-type gluten-free soy sauce
285ml/½ pint/1⅓ cups	water
1	clove garlic, crushed
1 heaped tbs	frozen peas
30g/1oz	ground almonds
1 heaped tbs	unflavoured yoghurt
1 level tsp	tomato purée (paste)
1 rounded tsp	brown sugar
2	hard-boiled eggs, peeled
	juice of ½ lemon

1   Gently fry the onion in the oil for 4 to 5 minutes without letting it brown.

2   Put in the ginger and curry powder and stir-fry for another minute. Take off the heat and put in the carrot, potato, soy sauce, water and garlic. Bring to the boil then simmer for 10 minutes, stirring from time to time. Put in the peas and continue cooking for another 5 minutes.

3   Mix the almonds, yoghurt, tomato purée and sugar in a cup. Add to the pan and stir in.

4   Add the eggs (whole) and heat gently for 5 minutes. (On no account let the curry boil.) Squeeze over the lemon juice, stir in and serve on a bed of boiled rice.

5   Serve with gluten-free chutney (*see page 115*), gluten-free poppadoms or chapattis (*see pages 37–38*) and side dishes of sliced fresh tomatoes, bananas, chopped spring onions (scallions), diced cucumber and more unflavoured yoghurt.

puddings

fruit on bread

serves one

1 portion	**stewed, sweetened fruit such as plums**
2 slices	**special gluten-free bread**
	sunflower oil for frying
	sugar for sprinkling

1 Heat the fruit and keep warm.
2 Fry the bread in shallow, hot oil on one side only. Put on to a warmed plate and top with fruit.
3 Sprinkle with sugar and serve.

variation   Any fruit from the plum family will do – damsons, greengages etc. (This is a very simple dish but really delicious. Other fruits such as apples are not half as good.)

pears in wine

serves one

1	**stewing pear**
1 glass	**red wine**
4 good pinches	**cinnamon**
	sugar to taste

1 Peel and quarter the pear and place it in a small saucepan.
2 Pour the wine over the pear and cook over a gentle heat until the pear is soft.
3 Sprinkle in the cinnamon and sugar to taste.
4 Serve warm or cold.

note to cooks   If the liquid reduces too much while the pear is cooking, then top up with water. (This can also be cooked in the oven in a small casserole.) For children, omit wine and use water instead with the finely grated zest of half a lemon.

crunchy date tart

pastry:

50g/2oz/¼ cup	**polyunsaturated soft margarine**
100g/4oz/½ cup	**ground rice**
75g/3oz/1 small	**finely grated apple**

filling:

100g/4oz/⅔ cup	**chopped cooking dates (or de-stoned eating dates)**
200ml/⅓ pint/¾ cup	**water**
40g/1½oz/¾ cup	**chopped nuts**
	sprinkling of sesame seeds

1 Preheat oven to 425°F/220°C/gas mark 7.
2 Put the dates into a small saucepan with the water and cook for a few minutes until they form a stiff paste. Leave to cool.
3 Use a fork to blend the pastry ingredients. Knead into one ball of dough.
4 Grease a pie plate and line it with the dough by pressing out evenly with the fingers.
5 Raise a slight edge all the way round.
6 Spread the date mixture over the pastry.
7 Sprinkle with the nuts and seeds, pressing them in slightly.
8 Bake on the top shelf for about 20 to 25 minutes.

orange caramel

serves one

1	**large orange**
1 heaped tsp	**sugar**
1 tbs	**water**

1 Pare off half the orange rind as thinly as you can and cut into strips.
2 Cut off the remaining rind and the white, bitter pith.
3 Slice the orange and place it in a serving dish.
4 Put the strips of rind into a small saucepan and sprinkle with the sugar. Add the water.
5 Heat while you stir until the sugar has melted.
6 Continue heating and stirring for a few minutes until you have a bubbly golden brown caramel. Pour this quickly over the orange.
7 Allow to cool, then chill in the fridge. Serve cold.

apricot tart with almonds

A refreshing pudding that can be served all year round, hot or cold.

makes six wedges

pastry:

50g/2oz/¼ cup	**polyunsaturated soft margarine**
100g/4oz/½ cup	**ground brown rice**
75g/3oz/1 small	**apple, grated**

filling:

150g/6oz/1 cup	**dried apricots**
2 heaped tsp	**sugar**
¼ litre/½ pint/1⅓ cups	**water, cold**
2 tsp	**fresh lemon juice**
25g/1oz/¼ cup	**almonds, shelled and chopped**

1   Preheat oven to 425°F/220°C/gas mark 7.
2   Pick over and wash the apricots before chopping them into small pieces.
3   Put into a saucepan with the sugar water and lemon juice. Bring to the boil and simmer until all the water has been absorbed.
4   Use a fork to blend the margarine, ground rice and apple. Knead until one ball of dough is formed.
5   Grease an enamel pie plate and put the dough in the centre. Flatten with the palm and fingers until it has spread evenly over the plate. Raise a slight edge all the way round with the fingers.
6   Spread the filling evenly over the pastry and sprinkle with the almonds.
7   Bake for 20 to 25 minutes on the top shelf and serve hot or cold in slices.

fruit tart

makes six wedges

50g/2oz/¼ cup	**polyunsaturated soft margarine**
100g/4oz/½ cup	**ground rice**
75g/3oz	**apple, finely grated**
4 portions	**stewing fruit**
200ml/⅓ pint/¾ cup or less	**water**
	sugar to taste

1 Preheat oven at 425°F/220°C/gas mark 7.

2 Use a fork to blend the margarine, ground rice and grated apple. Knead in the bowl until it forms one ball of dough.

3 Grease an enamel pie plate and put the dough in the centre. Flatten with the palm of the hand and press out to cover the plate evenly. Raise an edge all the way round with the fingers.

4 Bake on the top shelf for about 20 minutes.

5 Prepare the fruit and stew it in a little water. Sweeten to taste.

6 When the base has baked take it out of the oven and spread with the stewed fruit. Serve hot or cold, cut in wedges.

note to cooks   Blackberry and apple, plums, damsons etc. are particularly suitable for this recipe.

variation   Make the pastry base but bake for only 15 minutes. Take out of the oven and cover with a thin layer of apricot jam (jelly). Cover this with overlapping thin slices of apple. Sprinkle with sugar and put back in the oven for another 10 minutes. Serve as Apple Tart.

Make the pastry base and bake for the full time. Spread with raw sugar jam when it comes out of the oven. Serve warm or cold as Jam Tart.

Make the pastry base and bake for only 15 minutes. Take out of the oven and spread with treacle. Sprinkle with special wheat-free breadcrumbs and put back in the oven for another 10 minutes. Serve hot or cold as Treacle Tart.

apple amber

This useful sweet can be eaten straight from the oven or cold from the fridge. Serve to the whole family or to guests if you are entertaining. Alternatively, halve the recipe and serve to the gluten-free dieter, hot one day and cold the next.

serves four

500g/1 lb	**cooking apples, peeled, cored and chopped**
small knob/small pat	**butter**
	brown sugar to taste
1	**lemon, grated rind and juice**
2	**egg whites**
75g/3oz/⅓ cup	**caster (superfine) sugar**

1 Preheat the oven to 250°F/130°C/gas mark ½.
2 Put the apples in a pan with the butter and 1 tablespoon of water to prevent sticking. Cook gently until tender, then sweeten to taste with brown sugar.
3 Stir in the lemon rind and juice and then cook for another 5 minutes, stirring constantly. Transfer to an ovenproof pie dish.
4 Whisk the egg whites until very stiff. Fold in about 50g/2oz of the caster (superfine) sugar and pile lightly on top of the apple mixture. Sprinkle the remaining sugar over the meringue and bake for 30 to 40 minutes, until crisp on top.

carob pudding

serves two

¼ litre/½ pint/1⅓ cups	**water, cold**
2 slightly heaped tbs	**ground rice**
2 tsp	**vegetable oil**
3 heaped tsp	**sugar**
15g/½oz/1 tbs	**ground almonds**
1 heaped tsp	**carob powder**

1 Put the water and ground rice into a saucepan. Mix until smooth.
2 Add the oil and sugar and heat to boiling point. Cook while stirring for about 3 or 4 minutes, or until the pudding thickens.
3 Mix in the ground almonds and carob powder.
4 Serve hot or cold in 2 individual glasses.

variation   Sprinkle with flaked almonds before serving.

note to cooks   If you do not have carob powder in the cupboard, use a gluten-free brand of cocoa instead.

fruit and nut crumble

serves two

2 portions	**sweetened, stewed fruit – any kind in season**
1 tbs	**sunflower oil or similar**
15g/½oz/1 tbs	**ground almonds**
100g/4oz/½ cup	**ground rice**
3 tsp	**sugar**

1 Preheat oven to 425°F/220°C/gas mark 7.
2 Put the stewed fruit into a small ovenproof dish and flatten the top evenly.
3 Put all the other ingredients into a mixing bowl and rub in with the fingers until the mixture resembles very fine breadcrumbs.
4 Spoon the crumble evenly over the stewed fruit, covering it all over. Make a hole in the centre to let out the steam.
5 Bake for about 10 to 12 minutes, until golden brown.
6 Serve hot or cold.

baked bananas

A simple but delicious pudding.

serves four

4	**bananas, peeled and cut in half lengthways**
75g/3oz/½ cup	**sugar**
2	**small oranges, juice of**
25g/1oz/2½ tbs	**butter (optional)**

1   Preheat oven to 350°F/180°C/gas mark 4.

2   Put the halved bananas in an ovenproof dish.

3   Sprinkle with the sugar and pour the orange juice over the fruit.

4   Dot with the butter.

5   Bake for about 15 minutes on the top shelf.

6   Serve hot on warmed plates.

variation   Cut a passion fruit in half and squeeze over the bananas.

crème caramel

This is a useful sweet as it can be made in advance and served from the fridge. Take care not to let the caramel darken too much.

serves three

300ml/½ pint/1¼ cups	**milk**
40g/1½oz/3 tbs	**sugar**
1	**egg**
1	**egg yolk**
few drops	**vanilla flavouring**

caramel:

50g/2oz/¼ cup	**sugar**
2½ tbs	**water**

1 Preheat the oven to 325°F/160°C/gas mark 3.

2 Put the ingredients for the caramel into a small heavy-based pan. Heat gently, stirring, until the sugar has dissolved.

3 Increase the heat and allow to come to the boil. Cook without stirring until the caramel turns a light nut-brown colour – about 3 minutes. Pour immediately into 3 ovenproof ramekins or a heatproof dish.

4 Put the milk and sugar in a pan and stir over a moderate heat until it comes to the boil. Remove from the heat and pour through a fine strainer.

5 Beat the egg and egg yolk together in a bowl until thick and pale. Still beating, add the hot milk. Pour into a jug and stir in the vanilla flavouring.

6 Pour the milk and egg mixture into the prepared ramekins (or dish) through a fine strainer. Skim off any froth with a spoon.

7 Place the ramekins or dish in a deep baking tin (baking pan) and pour in enough boiling water to reach half way up the side of the ramekins or dish. Bake near the bottom of the oven for about 40 minutes or until set. Cool on a wire rack and then chill in the fridge.

8 When required, run a knife around the edge of the crème caramel. Put a serving plate upside-down on top, reverse the crème caramel and it will drop on to the plate.

note to cooks   Eat within 2 days.

three-fruit salad

1	eating apple or kiwi fruit (peeled)
1	orange, small
1	banana
1 small glass	unsweetened fruit juice (orange or pineapple)
	sugar

1 Prepare the fruits and cut into slices.
2 Pour the juice over the fruit and sprinkle with sugar to taste.

variation   Other fruits in season can be used, e.g. pineapple, peach, strawberries, raspberries, nectarines, tangerines etc. Do not use more than three types of fruit. Clear honey can be used instead of sugar. (This is the easiest of puddings and can be eaten all the year round. Leave the skin on the apple for extra fibre and colour.)

berry cream

serves three

¼ kilo/½ lb/2 cups	raspberries or blackberries
5 tbs	water
50g/2oz/⅓ cup	sugar
7g/¼oz/1 tsp	gelatine, dissolved in
2 tbs	cold water
150ml/¼ pint/⅔ cup	double (heavy) cream, lightly whipped

1 Pick over the raspberries and wash them.
2 Put the fruit into the blender with the water and sugar and blend to a *purée* (sauce).
3 Put through a sieve to remove pips.
4 Gently heat the soaked gelatine until completely dissolved, then stir into the *purée* (sauce).
5 Leave until it is just beginning to set, then fold in the cream.
6 Turn the mixture into individual glass dishes to set and serve chilled.

note to cooks Frozen raspberries, blackberries or summer fruits can be used.

eve's pudding

four servings

2	medium cooking apples
2 tbs	demerara sugar
	sponge bun batter *(see page 152)*

1 Preheat oven to 350°F/180°C/gas mark 4.

2 Grease a deep ovenproof pie dish.

3 Peel and core the apples. Cut into thin slices and arrange over the bottom of the dish. Sprinkle with the sugar.

4 Spread the bun mixture over the apples as evenly as you can.

5 Bake on a shelf above centre for 20 minutes until golden.

6 Serve hot with unflavoured yoghurt or gluten-free custard.

note to cooks   Make this a family pudding and serve to everybody.

apricot ice cream

serves three

150g/6oz/1 cup	**dried apricots**
1 tbs	**fresh lemon juice**
2	**egg whites**
75g/3oz/½ cup	**sugar**
150ml/¼ pint/⅔ cup	**double (heavy) cream, whipped**

1 Soak the apricots in water for about 2 hours.

2 Put the fruit into a small saucepan with enough water to cover and simmer gently for 20 minutes with the lid on.

3 Drain, saving 5 to 6 tablespoonsful of the liquid.

4 After cooling, put the cooked apricots, the reserved liquid and the lemon juice into the blender. Blend and cool completely.

5 Whisk the egg whites until stiff.

6 Gradually sprinkle in the sugar and whisk again.

7 Fold in the cream and apricot purée (sauce).

8 Turn the mixture into a freezer container. Cover, seal and freeze until the ice cream is solid.

9 Store in the freezer until required, and serve after transferring to the fridge for half an hour.

note to cooks   This is a useful recipe as it can be made all the year round.

baked apple

serves one

1	**cooking apple, large**
	water
	squeeze of fresh lemon juice
	sugar to taste

1   Preheat oven to 350°F/180°C/gas mark 4.

2   Wash the apple and, leaving it whole, cut a line around the middle. This will allow the flesh to expand during baking.

3   Cut out the core with an apple corer and discard.

4   Put the apple into an ovenproof dish and pour in about 150ml/¼ pint/⅔ cup of water.

5   Squeeze the lemon juice over the apple and sprinkle with sugar.

6   Bake for about 30 minutes on the top shelf.

7   Serve hot or cold.

note to cooks   For variations, stuff the apple cavity with sultanas, raspberries or blackberries.

blackcurrant dessert

serves one to two

1 slightly heaped tbs	**ground rice**
150ml/¼ pint/⅔ cup	**blackcurrants, stewed**
	sugar to taste
1 tsp	**sunflower oil**

1   Put all ingredients into a small saucepan and mix until smooth.
2   Heat to boiling point and cook, while stirring, for 2 minutes or until thick.
3   Leave to grow cold. Serve chilled from the fridge.

variation   Other fruit can be used e.g. stewed summer fruits, raspberries or apricots. You may need to purée the stewed fruit in a blender before using.

almond apple pudding

Serve this to the whole family to prove to them how good gluten-free food can be. Double the recipe to make 6 to 7 servings.

three generous servings

base:

75g/3oz/⅓ cup	brown sugar
125ml/4fl oz/½ cup	water
4	medium cooking apples, peeled, cored and cut into 8 wedges

topping:

40g/1½oz/3 tbs	butter
50g/2oz/¼ cup	caster (superfine) sugar
50g/2oz/½ cup	ground almonds
1	small lemon, juice and finely grated rind
1	egg, separated

1 Preheat the oven to 325°F/160°C/gas mark 3.

2 Put the brown sugar and water in a large saucepan and stir over a high heat until dissolved. Reduce the heat when it boils and continue to cook, without stirring, for about 4 minutes to make a syrup.

3 Add the apples to the pan, cover and cook gently for about 6 to 8 minutes, until tender.

4 Grease a sandwich tin (cake pan) large enough to hold the apples in one layer.

5 Beat the butter and caster (superfine) sugar until soft and light. Beat in the almonds, lemon juice and rind and egg yolk until well blended.

6 Whisk the egg white in a small bowl until it forms peaks. Use a metal spoon to fold it into the almond mixture.

7 Cover the base of the prepared tin (cake pan) with the apples, pouring over any remaining syrup. Spread with the topping and bake for about 20 minutes, until golden brown.

8 Cool in the tin (pan) for a few minutes, then serve with single (light) cream or on its own.

fruit brûlée

serves one

1 portion	**stewed fruit, sweetened to taste**
½ carton	**natural yogurt**
3 tsp	**sugar**

1 Put the stewed fruit into an individual-sized ovenproof dish.
2 Pour or spoon the yogurt over the fruit.
3 Sprinkle the sugar over the top of the yogurt.
4 Place under a hot grill until the sugar melts. Watch it carefully so as not to let it burn.
5 Serve right away.

real fruit jelly

serves three to four

400ml/¾ pint/2 cups	**pure fruit juice**
15g/½oz/1 tbs	**unflavoured gelatine crystals**
	sugar to taste

1 Put about one third of the fruit juice into a small saucepan and sprinkle in the gelatine crystals.
2 Stir well making sure there are no lumps.
3 Put over a very gentle heat and gradually bring to the boil, stirring all the time, to get out any lumps.
4 Add the rest of the fruit juice and stir well.
5 Put in the sugar to taste and stir until dissolved.
6 Pour into 3 to 4 individual glasses and leave to get cold.
7 Transfer to the fridge.
8 Serve cold, from the fridge, with a little single cream if desired.

note to cooks   For the fruit juice use any single juice or a combination of juices. Orange, liquidized strawberries, raspberries, cooked stoned prunes or dried apricots. Any left-over stewed fruit can also be used – blackberries, gooseberries, plums etc. Avoid pineapple and kiwi fruit as these will not set.

tarte du jour

A colourful treat for elevenses, tea time or dessert, this tart can be served confidently to everyone, not just the gluten-free dieter.

pastry:

50g/2oz/¼ cup	**gluten-free soft margarine**
100g/4oz/1 cup	**ground rice**
75g/3oz/¾ cup	**apple, finely grated**
pinch	**salt**

filling:

	Fresh fruit such as strawberries, raspberries or seedless grapes, stoned sweet cherries, peeled and sliced kiwi fruit or banana, or stoned and sliced peaches or nectarines.
2 tbs	**apricot jam**

1 Preheat the oven to 425°F/220°C/gas mark 7.

2 Put all the ingredients for the pastry into a bowl and blend with a fork until they form a dough.

3 Put the dough into the centre of an ovenproof plate or pie plate and gradually press it out with your fingers until the plate is evenly covered. Raise an edge all round by pinching between thumb and forefinger (flute it if you can).

4 Bake for 20 to 25 minutes until golden, then leave to cool on the plate.

5 When the base is completely cold, arrange the prepared fruit of your choice on top in concentric circles – all one fruit or a variety.

6 Put the apricot jam in a small pan with 1 tablespoonful of water and heat gently, stirring. Brush over the fruit with a pastry brush and leave to set.

7 Serve the tart with single cream for a special treat or just on its own.

tea time

fruit slices

left-over gluten-free pastry (from fruit tart etc.)

dried fruit

milk

sugar

1 Preheat oven to 425°F/220°C/gas mark 7.
2 Roll out the pastry and cut into 2 equal shapes.
3 Sprinkle one piece generously with dried fruit after brushing with milk.
4 Cover with the remaining piece of pastry and press the edges together.
5 Brush the top with milk and sprinkle with sugar.
6 Cut into fingers and place on baking sheet to bake for about 15 minutes. Serve freshly baked.

date and ginger cake

2 tbs	sunflower oil
50g/2oz/¼ cup	soft brown (molasses) sugar
1	egg, beaten
50g/2oz/½ cup	ground rice
25g/1oz/¼ cup	gluten-free cornflour (cornstarch)
25g/1oz/¼ cup	ground almonds
1 tsp	ground ginger
1	small eating apple, finely grated including skin
100g/4oz/⅔ cup	dates, stoned and chopped

1 Preheat the oven to 375°F/190°C/gas mark 5.
2 Put the oil, sugar, egg, ground rice and cornflour (cornstarch) into a bowl and beat until smooth.
3 Stir in the almonds, ginger, grated apple and dates. Mix well to distribute evenly.
4 Put the mixture into a greased and lined small loaf tin (loaf pan) and smooth the top with a knife.
5 Bake above the centre of the oven for about 45 to 50 minutes or until a skewer inserted in the centre comes out clean.
6 Cool in the tin (pan) for a few minutes, then turn out on to a wire rack to cool completely.
7 Wrap and store in an airtight container. Eat within 5 days. To freeze, wrap in individual slices.

almond fruit pastries

50g/2oz/¼ cup	**polyunsaturated soft margarine**
100g/4oz/½ cup	**ground brown rice**
1	**eating apple, large**
50g/2oz/⅓ cup	**brown sugar**
25g/1oz/¼ cup	**ground almonds**
few drops	**pure almond essence**
	sliced almonds for decoration

1 Preheat oven to 425°F/220°C/gas mark 7.

2 Blend margarine and ground rice using a fork.

3 Work in half the apple, grated, the sugar, ground almonds and flavouring. Knead until one ball of dough is formed.

4 Grease a baking sheet with margarine and put the dough in the middle. Flatten the dough out to a round shape by hand.

5 Cut the other half of the apple into thin slices and arrange these in the shape of a wheel, overlapping them slightly in the centre.

6 Sprinkle with a little more sugar and the sliced almonds.

7 Bake for 20 to 25 minutes until the pastry is cooked and the almonds toasted.

8 Allow to cool for a few minutes then serve, cut into wedges.

carrot cake

makes six slices

100g/3½oz	ground rice
30g/1oz	cornflour (cornstarch)
15g/½oz	gram (chickpea) flour
3 pinches	cream of tartar
1 good pinch	bicarbonate of soda
85g/3oz	sultanas
30g/2oz	polyunsaturated margarine, melted and cooled
85g/3oz/½ cup	finely grated carrot
30g/2oz	soft brown sugar
1 generous tbs	set honey
¼ level tsp	ground nutmeg
1 level tsp	ground ginger
1	egg, beaten

1   Preheat oven to 350°F/180°C/gas mark 4.

2   Mix the first 5 (dry) ingredients in a bowl.

3   Mix the sultanas, margarine, carrot, sugar, honey and spices in a second bowl.

4   Add the egg and mix again.

5   Put in the flour mixture and mix everything together to make a thick batter.

6   Spoon into a 15cm (6 in.) diameter cake tin, greased and floured with ground rice.

7   Bake for about 45 minutes on a shelf above centre. Test with a skewer to see if it is done. Leave in the tin for 5 minutes. Run a knife all round the edge and turn out onto a wire rack to cool

8   Eat within 2 days. Serve with confidence to everyone, not just the special dieter. Any left over can be individually wrapped and frozen for later use. Makes a good winter pudding served with gluten-free custard.

sponge buns

makes six

55g/2oz/⅓ cup	ground rice
15g/½oz	gram (chickpea) flour
30g/1oz	cornflour (cornstarch)
55g/2oz	caster sugar
1	egg, beaten
55g/2oz/¼ cup	polyunsaturated margarine
½ level tsp	cream of tartar
¼ level tsp	bicarbonate of soda
1 scant tsp	vanilla flavouring

1 Preheat oven to 375°F/190°C/gas mark 5.
2 Put the ground rice, gram flour, cornflour and sugar into a bowl. Mix well to combine.
3 Add remaining ingredients and mix/beat to a smooth cream.
4 Have ready a patty tin lined with 6 cake papers. Divide the mixture evenly between them and bake on the top shelf for 15 minutes until well risen and golden.
5 Put onto a wire rack to cool. Eat freshly baked or on the following day. Use stale buns for trifle.

chocolate sponge buns

Make as for Sponge Buns, adding 1 heaped tsp gluten-free cocoa and 1 tbs milk.

lemon shortbread

makes twelve small melt-in-the-mouth biscuits

50g/2oz/⅓ cup	**ground rice**
50g/2oz	**gluten-free cornflour (cornstarch)**
2 level tbs	**caster or soft brown sugar**
50g/2oz/¼ cup	**butter (straight from the fridge)**
rind of ½	**lemon**
2 tsp	**fresh lemon juice**

1 Preheat the oven to 425°F/220°C/gas mark 7.

2 In a bowl, blend the ground rice, cornflour (cornstarch) and sugar.

3 Add the butter cut into small pieces. Rub in well until the mixture resembles breadcrumbs.

4 Stir in the lemon rind and juice. Mix by hand to a firm dough. Knead for a minute until smooth.

5 Roll out using more cornflour (cornstarch) and cut into small shapes using cutters or a sharp knife.

6 Using a spatula, place on a greased baking sheet. Bake on the top shelf for about 10 minutes until golden and browning round the edges.

7 Take off the baking sheet with the spatula, being careful not to break them. Cool on a wire rack.

8 Store in an airtight container when cold and use within a week.

note to cooks   For variation, orange can be used instead of lemon. Crush biscuits into crumbs for use as a topping for plain, stewed apple to make a quick dessert.

sultana scones

makes eight small scones

30g/1oz	millet flour
30g/1oz	cornflour (cornstarch)
115g/4oz/⅔ cup	ground rice
¼ level tsp	bicarbonate of soda
½ level tsp	cream of tartar
1 slightly rounded tbs	sugar
30g/1oz	margarine
60g/2oz/⅓ cup	fresh mashed potato
60g/2oz	sultanas, chopped
	milk to bind

1 Preheat oven to 425°F/220°C/gas mark 7.
2 Mix the first 6 (dry) ingredients in a bowl.
3 Rub in the margarine and then the potato.
4 Sprinkle in the sultanas.
5 Stir in enough milk to bind and mix to a smooth, stiff dough. Divide into 6 pieces and shape each one into a scone.
6 Put onto a greased baking sheet and bake for 15 minutes on the top shelf.
7 When golden brown, take off the baking sheet and cool on a wire rack.
8 Serve split and buttered. Eat freshly baked. Any left over can be wrapped individually in cling film and split and toasted the following day.

celebration food

peach melba

serves four

2	ripe, sweet, fresh peaches
225g/8oz	fresh raspberries
55g/2oz	caster sugar
	homemade gluten-free vanilla ice cream *(see page 161)*
	gluten-free dessert wafers *(see page 160)*

1 Rub the peaches all over with the flat of a knife. Peel, halve and remove stones.
2 Rub the raspberries through a fine sieve, saving the juice in a bowl. Stir in the sugar.
3 For each serving, put 2 small scoops of ice cream into a sundae glass.
4 Place a peach half upside-down on top of the ice cream.
5 Spoon raspberry purée over the peach.
6 Serve on a saucer with a teaspoon and 2 wafers.

note to cooks Best assembled just before serving as the ice cream will melt quickly.

pavlova

four servings

meringue:

4	egg whites
2 pinches	salt
100g/4oz/½ cup	soft brown (molasses) sugar
1 tsp	gluten-free cornflour (cornstarch)
1 tsp	wine vinegar

filling:

150ml/¼ pint/⅔ cup	whipping cream (dairy)
1 slightly heaped tsp	icing (confectioner's) sugar
few drops	vanilla flavouring
225–275g/8–10oz	sweet fresh fruit, prepared *(see note overleaf)*

1 Preheat the oven to 300°F/150°C/gas mark 2.

2 Whisk the egg whites with the salt until they start to look glassy. Whisk in half the sugar, a little at a time, whisking well after each addition.

3 Mix the remaining sugar and cornflour (cornstarch) together. Use a metal spoon to fold them into the egg whites. Sprinkle the vinegar over the mixture and fold in gently.

4 Lightly grease a piece of greaseproof (wax) paper and dust with a little gluten-free cornflour (cornstarch). Place on a baking (cookie) sheet.

5 Use a spatula to spread out the meringue in a circle on the greaseproof (wax) paper, building it up more around the edge.

6 Bake for 60 to 70 minutes, then open the oven door wide and leave the meringue inside for about 15 minutes. Remove to a draught-free place until completely cold.

7 Whip the cream until thick, adding icing (confectioner's) sugar to taste and the vanilla. Chill in the fridge until required.

8 When almost ready to serve, carefully peel the paper off the base of the meringue. Put the meringue on a serving plate and spread the cream in the middle.

9 Arrange the fresh fruit on the top and serve cut into wedges.

note to cooks   Suitable fruits are raspberries, strawberries, slices of kiwi fruit, mango, pineapple, peaches or nectarines, and stoned cherries. A mixture of three or four of these is attractive.

Have the meringue, cream and fruit ready prepared and assemble at the last minute. A truly spectacular dessert!

christmas pudding

This is a rich golden pudding. Apart from its colour, there is very little difference between this one and the traditionally made type. Serve it confidently to the whole family. Make the day before eating.

makes eight helpings

2 tbs	lukewarm water
¼ litre/½ pint/1⅓ cups	orange juice
7g/¼oz	'fast action' Easyblend instant yeast
50g/2oz⅓ cup	brown sugar
25g/1oz/¼ cup	gram (chickpea) flour
150g/6oz/½ cup plus 2½ tbs	ground brown rice
½ tsp	each gluten-free mixed spice, cinnamon and nutmeg
50g/2oz/¼ cup	polyunsaturated soft margarine, melted
1	small eating apple
1	small carrot
325g/11oz/ 2 cups less 2½ tbs	dried mixed fruit
1	lemon, grated rind of
1	orange, grated rind of

1 Heat the water and fruit juice until lukewarm, using a small saucepan.

2 Add the yeast, sugar, soya flour, ground rice and spices and mix again.

3 Put in the margarine and grate in the apple and carrot. Beat until blended smoothly.

4 Add the fruit and rinds and mix well.

5 Grease a medium-sized pudding basin (1¼ litres/2½ pints/1½ US quarts) and spoon the mixture into this. Tie on a double greaseproof paper lid and make a string handle.

6 Lower the basin onto a large saucepan about one-third full with boiling water.

7 Have either a grid or 3 metal spoons in the bottom to keep the base of the pudding off the bottom of the pan. Put the lid on and steam for at least 1½ hours. (Top up with boiling water if the level goes down.)

8 Put a warm serving plate on top of the pudding after removing the paper lid. Hold firmly together and turn the bowl upside-down. Shake the pudding out onto the plate and serve hot.

note to cooks   If making a day ahead, steam for 1 hour. The following day, steam for ½ an hour.

dessert wafers

makes twelve delicate, crisp biscuits

45g/1½oz	ground rice
15g/½oz	cornflour (cornstarch)
1 tbs	caster sugar
½ tsp	vanilla flavouring
15g/½oz	polyunsaturated margarine
½	egg, beaten

1 Preheat oven to 400°F/200°C/gas mark 6.

2 Put the ground rice, cornflour, sugar and flavouring into a bowl. Mix well.

3 Add the margarine and rub in until mixture resembles breadcrumbs.

4 Stir in the egg and beat to a smooth cream.

5 Put teaspoons of the mixture onto a greased baking sheet, leaving plenty of space around each one for them to spread. With the back of the teaspoon spread the mixture out into fingers or circles.

6 Bake for about 8 minutes until golden brown around the edges. Put onto a wire rack to cool and crisp.

7 Serve freshly baked with gluten-free ice cream, sorbets or fruit salad.

note to cooks   Store any left over in an airtight container. Re-crisp in the oven for a minute when required. Eat within a week.

vanilla ice cream

Many commercial ice creams will contain gluten. Rather than shopping all over town to find a gluten-free brand, why not make your own?

six servings

285ml/½ pint/1⅓ cups	**milk**
½ tsp	**vanilla flavouring (or more to taste)**
1	**egg**
2	**egg yolks**
85g/3oz	**caster sugar**
285ml/½ pint/1⅓ cups	**double cream**

1 Pour the milk into a small saucepan and place over a gentle heat. Watch it carefully, removing from the heat just before it reaches boiling point. Stir in the flavouring and put aside to cool.

2 Put the egg, yolks and sugar into a bowl. Use a wooden spoon to beat to a pale cream.

3 Stir in the cooled milk. Mix well and put through a fine mesh sieve into a clean bowl.

4 Have ready a saucepan one quarter full of boiling water. Set the bowl over it and let the pan simmer to provide a very gentle heat. Stir until it thickens and will coat the back of a spoon. Pour into a clean bowl and leave to cool.

5 Lightly whip the cream. Fold in the cooled mixture. Thoroughly mix (don't beat) and spoon into an ice cube tray. Cover and put into the freezer.

6 When slushy and forming ice around the edge, turn into a bowl and whisk thoroughly. Put back into the ice cube tray and freeze until firm.

celebration brownies

makes sixteen

140g/5oz	polyunsaturated margarine
200g/7oz	plain gluten-free chocolate, chopped coarsely
2	eggs, beaten
140g/7oz	soft brown sugar
¼ tsp	vanilla flavouring
85g/3oz	cornflour (cornstarch)
30g/1oz	ground rice
pinch	salt
2 good pinches	bicarbonate of soda
¼ level tsp	cream of tartar
115g/4oz	skinned, toasted hazelnuts, coarsely chopped
	icing sugar for finishing

1   Preheat oven to 350°F/180°C/gas mark 4.

2   Prepare a 17cm (7 in.) square, shallow baking tin. Grease and line with greaseproof paper, extending 5cm (2 in.) over the sides of the tin.

3   Place a bowl over a pan of hot water. Put the margarine into the bowl with 55g/2oz of the chocolate. Leave to melt.

4   Use a large bowl to mix the eggs, sugar and flavouring. Pour in the melted margarine/chocolate mixture, sift in the cornflour and sprinkle in the ground rice, salt, bicarbonate of soda and cream of tartar. Fold/stir gently (don't beat) until all the ingredients are thoroughly mixed.

5   Stir in the remaining chocolate and the nuts.

6   Pour into the prepared tin and use the back of a metal spoon to spread it out evenly.

7   Bake for about 30 minutes on a shelf above centre. When the sides begin to shrink away from the tin, take out of the oven. Leave in the tin to cool on a wire rack.

8   Peel off paper and cut into 16 squares. Dust lightly with icing sugar and serve freshly baked as a treat.

marzipan

Store-bought marzipan is not usually gluten-free.

225g/8oz/2 cups	**ground almonds**
100g/4oz/½ cup	**caster sugar**
100g/4oz/1¼ cups	**icing (confectioner's) sugar, plus extra for dusting**
½	**egg, beaten**
1 tsp	**fresh lemon juice**
few drops	**almond essence**

1 Put the ground almonds and sugars into a bowl and stir to combine.
2 Make a well in the centre and put in the lemon juice, almond favouring and egg. Knead into a ball.
3 Roll out the marzipan on a board dusted with icing sugar. Handle it as little as possible or it will be too sticky.

chocolates

Make small balls of marzipan (*above*). Spear with a darning needle and dip into gluten-free chocolate melted in a bowl placed over a pan of hot water. Coat all over and leave to set on baking parchment.

sherry trifle

Use a sponge bun for the trifle base *(see page 152).*

one serving

1	**gluten-free sponge bun**
1 tbs	**red jam**
1 scant tbs	**sherry**
2 tbs	**sliced canned peaches or apricots, with a little juice**
about 4 tbs	**gluten-free custard (use appropriate custard powder or**
	gluten-free cornflour (cornstarch) and vanilla flavouring)
about 2 tbs	**whipped cream (dairy)**
1	**glacé (candied) cherry, washed**
a few	**toasted almonds**

1 Slice the bun in two and sandwich together with the jam. Break into pieces, place in a glass dish and spoon over the sherry.
2 Arrange the peaches or apricots on top and spoon over a little juice.
3 Cover with the custard and leave to set.
4 Spread the whipped cream on top, sprinkle with the almonds and put the cherry in the centre.

note to cooks   Make sure the cake base is nicely moistened with the jam, sherry and fruit juice.

pear and chocolate trifle

Make as for Sherry Trifle but use chocolate buns for the base and canned pears for the fruit. Top with gluten-free chocolate blancmange instead of custard and grate gluten-free chocolate to sprinkle on top of the cream. Place the cherry on last.

savoury straws

25g/1oz/1 tbs	**cold, boiled mashed potato**
15g/½oz/1 tbs	**polyunsaturated soft margarine**
pinch	**sea salt**
50g/2oz/¼ cup	**ground brown rice**
1 heaped tsp	**onion or shallot, very finely chopped**

1   Preheat oven to 425°F/220°C/gas mark 7.

2   Beat the potato to a cream with the margarine.

3   Gradually add the salt and ground rice and combine with a fork.

4   Put in the onion and mix well into one ball of dough. (If it too dry, add a little water.)

5   Press out by hand on a surface flavoured with ground rice.

6   Cut into fingers with a sharp knife and use a spatula to put them on a greased baking sheet.

7   Bake for about 8 to 10 minutes. (Do not overbake or they will be too crisp.)

gluten-free for children

Children on a special diet will need extra care and understanding. A sense of belonging to a group around their own age is one of the essentials of childhood, together with their own ideas of appropriate clothes, shoes, toys and behaviour. It is not a world that the adult completely understands as it is constantly undergoing change, but it needs to be taken into consideration. The other important element is food.

A child's instincts are geared to eating in order to survive and grow. Whereas adults are often trying to reduce or at least not to increase in weight, children need extra food to grow and develop into adults. Hunger plays an important part in the life of every child so a diet which is restricted in some way is particularly hard for the coeliac/allergic child.

The sense of belonging to a group can be damaged by having to eat different food which other children might see as inferior. If the group and family perceive the child to be weak and sick, this becomes obvious to the child and the sense of belonging is poor. Adults can help with their *attitude*. A special child deserves a special diet is a better concept than a sick child is a nuisance requiring different food from the rest of the family.

Sharing food is important. If the child's food is enviable it can be served to the whole family on some days. This does wonders for the 'belonging factor' and is a boon to the cook.

One of the dangers of a special diet is the child being tempted by friends or relatives into eating inappropriate food. This will probably feature junk snack foods, drinks and confectionery, all of which may contain gluten, the invisible danger. The child must be taught how to handle the situation. Make a large bag of Snax (*see page 171*), enough for the child and extra for friends. (Envy is easier to deal with than scorn.)

Encouraging children to eat fruit instead of sweets is a good policy. A nice red apple, polished up with a clean tea towel so that it shines, is quite tempting. Bananas, pure fruit juices and plain toasted nuts will always be popular, particularly if varied day to day.

For children of school age on a gluten-free diet, contact the head teacher to explain the situation and what the problems are. It may be safer, and less trouble for the staff, to send the child to school with a gluten-free packed lunch rather than suffer the difficulties of mass catering. It will depend entirely on how the child's diet is dealt with but no parent should delegate the responsibility completely to the school staff who are unlikely to have knowledge of the problem unless they have had first-hand experience.

Older children should be able to take responsibility for themselves. Remember, special children need a special diet, and by sticking to the diet there can be freedom from unpleasant symptoms.

What about children's parties or tea time at a friend's house? Some mums go to pieces at the thought of preparing special food as well as ordinary food and are much happier when the special food arrives with the guest.

Children will enjoy many of the recipes in this book, but for a treat, here are some recipes designed especially with children in mind.

snax

Snack nibbles for treats or as part of a lunchbox are a problem as most commercial ones contain gluten and come into the junk food category. Bake your own healthier version and make up into little bags to eat away from home. For adults, these nibbles can also be served at dinner or at drinks parties.

makes 125g/4oz, about eighty nibbles

45g/1½oz	**ground rice**
15g/½oz	**cornflour (cornstarch)**
15g/½oz	**gram (chickpea) flour**
2 good pinches	**salt**
1 level tbs	**finely grated Parmesan cheese**
20g/¾oz	**polyunsaturated margarine**
60g/2oz/⅓ cup	**mashed potato**
1 tbs	**water (if required)**
	more cornflour for handling

1   Preheat oven to 375°F/190°C/gas mark 5.
2   Put the rice, cornflour, gram flour, salt and cheese into a bowl. Mix well to combine.
3   Add the margarine and rub in until the mixture resembles crumbs.
4   Put in the potato and pull the mixture together to make 1 ball, adding the water. Knead for a minute in the bowl.
5   Break off about ¼ of the dough. Using cornflour, roll into a sausage about 15cm (6 in.) long. With a sharp knife, cut off about 20 thin slices and put onto a greased baking sheet. Continue until all the dough has been used.
6   Bake on the top shelf for about 10 minutes until golden. Leave to cool on the baking sheet. When completely cold, store in an airtight container. Eat within a week.

mini pizzas

Make for a snack and serve cut into wedges.

makes one medium or two small pizzas

170g/6oz	pizza dough *(see page 33)*
3	canned, peeled plum tomatoes, chopped or
2	fresh tomatoes, sliced
2 or 3	kinds of vegetable *(see page 173)*
1	small clove garlic, crushed
3	fresh basil leaves, torn into small pieces or
½ tsp	dried basil
1 heaped tbs	finely grated, tasty Cheddar cheese for topping
5	black olives, halved and de-stoned

1   Preheat oven to 425°F/220°C/gas mark 7.

2   Put the dough on an ovenproof plate. Press out with the fingers to a circle about 15cm (6 in.) in diameter. Raise an edge all round.

3   Cover with tomato.

4   Arrange your choice of vegetables on top.

5   Distribute the garlic, putting small dabs on the vegetables. Scatter the herb over, sprinkle on the cheese and distribute the olives.

6   Bake on the top shelf for 15 minutes until the pastry is golden and the cheese melted and bubbling. Eat hot off the baking plate.

vegetable topping suggestions:

- ½ courgette (zucchini), thinly sliced
- ¼ pepper, de-seeded and chopped
- 1 heaped tbs frozen peas (defrosted)
- ½ stick celery, chopped
- 3 button mushrooms, chopped or sliced
- 2 heaped tbs gluten-free baked beans, drained

note to cooks   For a party, cut into small wedges and serve on folded paper napkins or small plates. Some children will prefer pizza without the herbs and olives.

lemon drops

makes twelve biscuits

45g/1½oz	**ground rice**
15g/½oz	**maize flour**
15g/½oz	**gram (chickpea) flour**
15g/½oz	**potato flour**
30g/1oz	**polyunsaturated margarine**
1 slightly rounded tbs	**caster sugar**
1	**egg, beaten**
	finely grated rind of ½ lemon

1 Preheat oven to 425°F/220°C/gas mark 7.
2 Mix the first 5 ingredients in a bowl.
3 Rub in the margarine and sprinkle in the sugar.
4 Add the egg and rind. Mix to a sticky wet paste.
5 Using 2 teaspoons, put small mounds of the mixture onto a greased baking sheet, leaving plenty of space around each one to allow for spreading.
6 Bake for 10 minutes on the top shelf until brown round the edges.
7 Loosen with a spatula after 5 minutes and put onto a wire rack to cool. Store in an airtight container. Eat within a week. The biscuits can be re-crisped in a hot oven for a minute if necessary.

chocolate drops

Make as for Lemon Drops but omit lemon. Add 1 heaped teaspoon cocoa and a little milk.

alphabet biscuits

Use the Lemon Drops recipe. When cool, ice letters of the alphabet or initials on the biscuits with water icing. These go down well with children at a party or for everyday special 'attention'. The feelgood factor scores high with these!

jelly trifle

one serving

1	gluten-free sponge bun *(see page 152)*
2 tbs	sliced fresh or canned peaches or canned apricots
4–5 tbs	hot, liquid fruit jelly
	Real Fruit Jelly *(see page 143)*

1 Break up the bun and put it in a glass dish.
2 Arrange the fruit on top of the sponge. Spoon over the jelly and leave to set.
3 Place in the fridge and serve within 48 hours, with cream or gluten-free ice cream if liked.

coping generally

packed meals

Don't fall into the trap of putting up with packed meals that are largely stodge. Try to imitate a meal eaten at home for balance. Soup can be taken in a vacuum flask for instance. Salads can be packed in a screw-top jar with another small jar containing dressing to put on just before eating. Pack slices of cold meat between small sheets of greaseproof paper. Cheese can be grated and put into a small plastic container to be sprinkled over salad.

Instead of bread, slice cold cooked potatoes and put into a plastic box. Bananas, apples, pears and grapes make perfect snacks but don't forget dried apricots, raisins and sultanas (golden seedless raisins) as well as nuts of all kinds.

Try to make the basis of the packed meal a protein one – meat, fish, eggs, cheese or nuts. The energy part of the meal, gluten-free bread and potatoes, should not be too much in evidence, nor should you pack too much sweet and sugary food. A slice of rich fruit cake is much better than chocolate bars or stodgy biscuits. If fruit becomes boring try fresh fruit juice with an ice cube in a vacuum flask for a cooling summer drink.

It isn't a bad idea to keep a note of just what you put into packed meals if you have to cope with this every day. You can then avoid too much repetition.

The secret really is always to try to make the special dieter's food enviable and this applies just as much to food you are sending out from home as the food you put on the table.

general list of gluten-free items

All kinds of cheeses (plain)
  – not spreads

Bacon

Black treacle

Brandy

Brown or white rice

Butter

Canned fruit

Chocolate (good makes),
  plain, without fillings*

Chopped peel and cherries

Cider

Coffee (pure)

Cornflakes*

Cream (dairy)

Crisps (plain)

Cut mixed peel

Desiccated coconut

Fish (fresh, uncoated),
  canned in oil or water
  (not sauce)

Flaked rice

Fruit (fresh, canned or dried)

Fruit juices (unsweetened)

Ground brown rice

Ground white rice

Herbs, fresh or dried

Honey (pure)

Jam (jelly)

Margarine (without
  wheatgerm oil)

Marmalade

Meat (fresh or frozen, plain)

Milk (fresh or dried)

Natural yogurts

Nuts (plain)

Oils (except wheatgerm oil)

Rice Krispies (UK)*

Sherry

Spices (pure)

Squashes

Sugar

Syrup

Tapioca

Tea

Vegetables (fresh, canned in
  water or frozen, plain)

Wine

Wine vinegar

* indicates ingredients must be checked before using

balancing your diet

The average Western diet has many faults – far too much fat, sugar and salt; too little of fresh vegetables, fruit and fibre-rich foods; too many over-processed junk foods etc. Try to avoid these dietary pitfalls and balance your diet in this way to rectify matters:

15% fats, oils (including cheese), nuts and seeds
20% meat, fish and eggs
45% fresh vegetables and fruit (including a green leafy vegetable daily)
20% special gluten-free bakery items, including bread

The basic food in a gluten-free diet is not balanced in the same way as a diet where gluten-containing foods are staples. Here are the basic food values in a gluten-free diet:

Protein – meat, fish, eggs, nuts, dairy produce
Fat – cheese, cooking oils, fish and meat, nuts and seeds
Carbohydrate – rice, potatoes, bananas, special bread and bakery items, sugar
Fibre – soya bran, rice bran, root vegetables, dried fruits
Vitamins and minerals – fresh vegetables and fruit

A wide variety of fresh foods should give you all the nourishment you need for a healthy diet. However, food supplements (vitamins and minerals) can be taken if they are felt to be necessary. These should also be gluten-free (specially formulated) like the rest of the diet. Check with your medical practitioner or pharmacist.

coping at home

Some people can take the situation of having a special dieter in the family seemingly in their stride. Others are not able to cope quite as well. The dieter eats the wrong things and never seems to be really well. Perhaps the secret is to be really organized about it and if possible to get the full co-operation of the dieter.

Make sure your special store-cupboard is always stocked up. Teach the dieter to cook for him or herself if at all possible so that they will be able to cope with their own food in an emergency or just to give the usual cook a bit of a holiday.

If you can prepare things that the whole family can enjoy then so much the better – this saves preparing two kinds of food. Try to present the special food attractively and make it appetizing. Whatever you do, don't make the special dieter feel a burden. This can lead to emotional problems within the family unit.

Avoid a dull routine of cooking the same old recipes. There are several books available on gluten-free cooking now and this kind of exclusion diet isn't the dreary type it used to be, thank goodness. There are a variety of gluten-free diet foods available too. Try your local health store for these.

Don't forget, foods made from *wheat starch* are likely to contain gluten even though labelled 'gluten-free'.

holidays

If going on a self-catering holiday you can take with you a variety of recipes made up, as far as possible, for cooking and baking during the holiday. For instance, you can make up a few of the bread blends (dry ingredients only) and take the yeast with you to bake as you need them. (Add the other ingredients just before baking.) A rich fruit cake is a good standby and will keep a week at least. Biscuits can be made too and kept in an air-tight tin. Crumble topping can be made up and kept in the refrigerator (if there is one) and used as required.

If the holiday is not self-catering then you will have to take some of the special foods you know you won't be able to obtain. Again, a rich fruit cake is a good standby, also biscuits.

If possible, notify the catering manager or equivalent of the place where you plan to stay that you have someone in your party who is on a special diet. This can avoid misunderstandings with the serving staff who can take offence at someone whom they think is just plain finicky and a nuisance. Very often it comes as a pleasant surprise that staff will take no end of trouble to make sure the special diet is accommodated. However, do not take this for granted and have some standby items just in case. **As a general rule, catering staff, however well qualified, have no knowledge of catering for a special diet.**

One golden rule – never go on holiday without your diet food list; and remember, millions of people cope daily with a special diet so you are not alone. Don't think of it as a terrible problem, just get yourself organized and take it in your stride.

index